CRYSTAL
PRESCRIPTIONS

Volume 5

The A-Z guide to Space Clearing,
Feng Shui and Psychic Protection
Crystals

CRYSTAL
PRESCRIPTIONS

Volume 5

The A-Z guide to Space Clearing,
Feng Shui and Psychic Protection
Crystals

Judy Hall

Author of the best-selling
The Crystal Bible series

BOOKS

Winchester, UK
Washington, USA

JOHN HUNT PUBLISHING

First published by O-Books, 2016
O-Books is an imprint of John Hunt Publishing Ltd., 3 East St., Alresford,
Hampshire SO24 9EE, UK
office@jhpbooks.com
www.johnhuntpublishing.com

For distributor details and how to order please visit the 'Ordering' section on our
website.

ISBN: 978 1 78535 457 1
978 1 78535 458 8 (ebook)

A CIP catalogue record for this book is available from the British Library.

Design: Stuart Davies

UK: Printed and bound by CPI Group (UK) Ltd, Croydon, CR0 4YY
US: Printed and bound by Thomson-Shore, 7300 West Joy Road, Dexter, MI 48130

We operate a distinctive and ethical publishing philosophy
in all areas of our business, from our global network of
authors to production and worldwide distribution.

Volumes in this series:

Crystal Prescriptions
The A–Z guide to over 1,200 symptoms and their healing crystals
ISBN: 978-1-90504-740-6 (Paperback) £7.99 $15.95

Crystal Prescriptions volume 2
The A–Z guide to over 1,250 conditions and their new
generation healing crystals
ISBN: 978-1-78279-560-5 (Paperback) £8.99 $14.95

Crystal Prescriptions volume 3
Crystal solutions to electromagnetic pollution and geopathic stress.
An A–Z guide.
ISBN: 978-1-78279-791-3 (Paperback) £8.99 $14.95

Crystal Prescriptions volume 4
The A–Z guide to the chakra balancing crystals and kundalini
activation stones
ISBN: 978-1-78535-053-5 (Paperback) £10.99 $17.95

Crystal Prescriptions volume 5
Space clearing, Feng Shui and Psychic Protection.
An A-Z guide.
ISBN: 978-1-78535-457-1 (Paperback) £12.99 $19.95

Crystal Prescriptions volume 6
Crystals for ancestral clearing, soul retrieval, spirit release and karmic
healing. An A-Z guide.
ISBN: 978-1-78535-455-7 (Paperback) £13.99 $19.95

Crystal Prescriptions volume 7
The A-Z Guide to Creating Crystal Essences for Abundant
Well-Being, Environmental Healing and Astral Magic
ISBN: 978-1-78904-052-4 (Paperback) £17.99 $29.95

CONTENTS

Acknowledgements

My thanks go to all those who have taught me about the need for psychic protection over the years, those who opened my eyes to the effects of geopathic stress, and those who introduced me to Feng Shui. And, of course, to the crystal oversouls that have provided solutions. Blessings to you all.

Disclaimer
The information given in this directory is in no way intended to be a substitute for treatment by a medical practitioner. Further assistance should be sought from a suitably qualified crystal healer. Healing can be defined as bringing the body, emotions, mind and spirit back into balance. It does not imply a cure.

Introduction: Safe and Sound

Just as treasures are uncovered from the earth, so virtue appears from good deeds, and wisdom appears from a pure and peaceful mind. To walk safely through the maze of human life, one needs the light of wisdom and the guidance of virtue.
Buddha

For many people, crystals are divine light that has crystallised and taken on form. They carry virtue and wisdom within them. Crystals help you to find your own inner light, your divine being. A connection that instils confidence and a feeling of safety knowing that you are an eternal soul that happens to be on a human journey. Some people call that inner light God, others Source, Spirit, the crystal oversouls, the divine or enlightenment. Whatever name you give it, once you are attuned to it, it provides you with a sense of being protected by a greater power. A power of which you are an integral part, not an outsider. And that light takes you beyond the cares and worries of everyday into a quiet peaceful *sacred* space within your Self. Over the last thirty-five years I've written several books on space clearing and psychic protection. Each time I hoped I'd said everything that needed to be said. And then something else would come along. New challenges, new crystals, new ways of looking at things. But never before have I gathered together all the protective crystal possibilities into a directory such as this one. Whether you need to create a safe space for everyday living or meditation, or craft an oasis of calm in a buzzing work environment, or protect your home in a crime-ridden area, crystals will assist you. You'll be able to work in harmony with the Feng Shui bagua to harmonize your home, attract abundance and enhance all areas of your life. You'll find crystals to ghostbust, to clear curses no matter how far back in your ancestral line, to remove spirit attachments, and to retrieve lost soul parts. Crystals that help you to strengthen your aura, create an interface between you and the outside world, and repel psychic invasion are also to be found here. Crystals such as Shungite and Black Tourmaline absorb and entrap – what I would call block – detrimental energies. Other crystals transmute energy turning the potentially toxic and negative into the beneficial and positive:

Cancellation or generation of positive energy by negative energy and vice versa is so often brought up by very serious physicists (e.g. A. Guth, AV Filippenko) as the argumentation for the possibility of the generation of our universe out of "nothing", that I hardly dare to question this. As an example or metaphor for it is most often used the so called cancellation of (so called positive) kinetic energy by the (so called negative) gravitational energy. But, to me, energy will never be cancelled, it will always be exchanged. https://www.physicsforums.com/threads/negative-energy-versus-positive-energy.126045/

The writer of that quote is a physicist, and physicists name their energies somewhat differently to crystal healers. But we often forget that you cannot just negate and cancel energy, energy doesn't die. It has to be transformed or transmuted. Even when it is, apparently, captured within a blocking stone such as Shungite, it does transform. Equally when we cleanse a stone this is in effect what we are doing with the energy. The toxic dross doesn't just disappear. It is transmuted. A process more akin to alchemy than rigid orthodox science – which, we must never forget, grew out of alchemical roots aeons ago.

Getting to grips with the basics

You may find some material here that you have read before. The basics remain the same but are reiterated in case this is the first of my books that you have picked up. But even if you are highly experienced, it never hurts to remind yourself of essential working practices such as cleansing, programming and grounding yourself. Other information is equally vital. My *Crystal Prescriptions volume 3* is a comprehensive guide to counteracting electromagnetic frequencies and geopathic stress, for instance. But nevertheless you'll find these topics briefly referred to here – in less detail. Just the essential basics. But you can't keep your space clear without knowing something of the topic. The same can be said for ancestral clearing, soul work and karmic healing. *Crystal Prescriptions volume 6* focuses specifically on those areas, but this volume too gives you first aid measures in case the ancestors or your own karmic past are interfering with your protection and well-being in this life.

Before you begin: please remember!

If you don't cleanse your crystals regularly even they may be detrimental as they absorb and then, when overstuffed, give off negative energies.

Cleaning your crystals is simple if you choose tumbled stones, rugged chunks or single points. You simply have to hold them under running water for a few minutes and, preferably, put them out in the sun and possibly the moon to recharge. White crystals are particularly fond of moonlight. Or, you can put them on to a large Quartz cluster or Carnelian to reboot. You can also use salt water to cleanse robust stones. If you use crystal clusters or stones that are fragile or dissolve, such as Selenite, the crystals need placing in raw brown rice overnight (see page 22). My favourite crystal cleansing tool is Petaltone Clear2Light and Zl4. One drop and it's done (see Resources). The reason that crystals sometimes don't work for people, even when they've identified exactly the right one, is that they forget to ask. So, once the crystal has been cleaned and energetically recharged, hold it in your hands and ask that it work for your highest good to protect you. You can be specific, or you can allow the natural intelligence of the crystal to recognize what you need. Once again, more details follow.

Over to you

The most effective thing you can do to protect yourself is to take responsibility for your own thoughts, feelings, actions and environment and the state of your own soul. To become your authentic self. The way that you choose to do this is up to you. This book offers you a choice of crystal assistants and ways to use them. Pick the ones that resonate best with you.

Essential Information

This section gives you essential guidance and background information that will assist you to get the most out of your crystals. Do please read through it even if you are familiar with crystal working. Crystals are powerful tools that pick up and amplify your thoughts and could well attract to you exactly what you are trying to avoid. They should be treated with respect.

Finding Your Prescription

Most entries in this directory offer a choice of crystals to assist a challenge, condition or issue. You may find that you are instinctively drawn to a particular stone and it may be one that you already have in your collection. If so, try this one first. Alternatively, the best way to select your crystals and to identify where to place them is to dowse for them (see page 16). While all the stones listed in the directory could potentially help you, selecting the right crystal is crucial if you are to obtain maximum benefit and the fastest relief or most effective harmonizing and/or blocking. As everyone has their own unique vibration and auric field, different crystals will be required even though a situation may appear on the surface to be exactly the same. Some crystals have a much finer vibration than others, working from the etheric to adjust the physical, and some work purely at a physical level so you may need to use a series of crystals or combine them within a grid.

Use the innate ability of your intuitive body-mind connection to tune into subtle vibrations and to influence your hands. A focused mind, trust in the process, carefully worded questions and a clear intent will support your dowsing and your healing.

Framing your question

Framing your question Framing your question with precision is essential if you are to achieve the most beneficial result especially if you are trying to keep yourself and your space safe. Your questions need to be unambiguous and capable of a straight 'yes' or 'no' answer if you are dowsing. Sit quietly for a few moments, bringing your focus away from the outside world and quietening your mind. Word your question carefully. You need to be specific. If you are finger dowsing (see page 18), ask: "Is [name of crystal] the best and most appropriate crystal to protect my energies at this time?" If you are pendulum dowsing (see page 16), ask: "Please show me the best and most appropriate crystal to protect me now." Asking "Why do I need psychic protection?" would be complex but could reveal the underlying cause, which may need to be treated with different crystals. If you are subject to constant bombardment by other

14

people's thoughts for instance, in addition to putting up a 'keep out' notice crystal, you will need to repair any underlying 'faulty' chakra or auric field problems too. So always ask, is there any underlying cause, and work to heal that. Finger or pendulum dowsing will also assist in selecting exactly the right place to position your crystal when creating an energetic net to absorb and transmute negative energies. You can also dowse to ascertain the best shape to use for a grid (see page 19).

Dowsing

Dowsing quickly identifies the right crystal for you. It is an excellent way to locate geopathic stress lines when space clearing or to demonstrate chakra blockages. You can either use a pendulum for this purpose or finger, body or rod dowse (see page 19). Rods move inward and cross, or move outwards, as they reach a geopathic stress line or enter an area of electromagnetic smog or other environmental disturbance. Pendulums spin wildly or sluggishly according to how a chakra is functioning. Muscle testing can also rapidly pinpoint the right crystal for you. There are several methods of dowsing so try them all until you find the one that works best for you and then practise to refine your technique. You will need to establish your yes and no signal if using a pendulum (see below). Dowsing for solutions works best in an energetically clear space.

Pendulum dowsing

If you are familiar with pendulum dowsing, use the pendulum in your usual way. If you are not, this skill is easily learned. Crystal pendulums are useful for this but wooden or metal ones can also be used.

To pendulum dowse

To pendulum dowse, hold your pendulum between the thumb and forefinger of your most receptive hand with about a hand's length of chain hanging down to the pendulum – you will soon learn what is the right length for you. Wrap the remaining chain around your fingers so that it does not obstruct the dowsing.

You will need to ascertain which is a 'yes' and which a 'no' response. Some people find that the pendulum swings in one direction for 'yes' and at right angles to that axis for 'no', while others have a backwards and forwards swing for one reply, and a circular motion for the other. A 'wobble' of the pendulum may indicate a 'maybe' or that it is not appropriate to dowse at that time, or that the wrong question is being asked. In which case, ask if it is appropriate, and if the answer is 'yes', check that you are framing the question in the correct way. If the pendulum stops completely it is usually inappropriate to ask at that time.

You can ascertain your particular pendulum response by holding the pendulum over your knee and asking: "Is my name [correct name]?" The direction that the pendulum swings will indicate 'yes'. Check by asking: "Is my name [incorrect name]?" to establish 'no'. Or, you can programme in 'yes' and 'no' by swinging the pendulum in a particular direction a few times, saying as you do: "This is 'yes'," and swinging it in a different direction to programme in 'no'.

Once yes or no is established, simply place your

finger on a crystal, or its name, and ask "Is this crystal beneficial for me?" You may identify several possible crystals and need to refine the answer – see Framing your question, page 14.

Finger dowsing

Finger dowsing answers 'yes' and 'no' questions quickly and unambiguously, and may be done unobtrusively in situations where a pendulum might provoke unwanted attention. This method of dowsing works particularly well for people who are kinaesthetic, that is to say their body responds intuitively to subtle feelings, but anyone can learn to finger dowse.

To finger dowse

To finger dowse, hold the thumb and first finger of your right hand together (see illustration). Loop the thumb and finger of your left hand through to make a 'chain'. Ask your question clearly and unambiguously – you can speak it aloud or keep it within your mind. Now pull

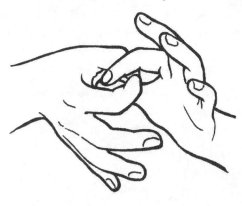

gently but firmly. If the chain breaks, the answer is usually 'no'. If it holds, the answer is usually 'yes' – but check by asking your name in case your response is reversed.

To rod dowse

You can use purpose-made dowsing rods, y-shaped hazel twigs or cut wire coat hangers into right-angled shapes to find detrimental energy lines. Hold the rods loosely in your hands, fingers curled inwards to make a holder, and slowly walk forwards across a room or site. Ask to be shown where the lines of disturbance are. The rods will move or twitch when you reach the front edge and move back to straight when you pass beyond it.

Body dowsing

As bodies are extremely sensitive to changing vibrations you could use your hands or feet to dowse your space.

To body dowse

- If you are using your hands, rub your hands together briskly to open your palm chakras.
- Extend your hands forwards with your palms turned up and facing out.
- Walk slowly and when you reach the line or area of disturbed energy it will feel as though you are pushing against an invisible wall.
- Your feet may tingle if the space is beneficial, or your knees go weak and feel like you are walking

through treacle if the space is harmful. Feet may also tingle when you reach a geopathic stress or beneficial ley line.

• Similarly, if you hold your palm down over a chakra and it is blocked, it will feel lifeless or sticky. If it is whirling too fast, you will feel a strong and uncomfortable buzzing in your palm.

You can use your palms or your fingertips to choose your crystals too. A crystal that will work for you or your space will feel lively, tingly as you pick it up. Place it in your space and, if your hand then feels calm as you place it, this is the crystal for you.

Muscle testing

Another method that utilises body dowsing is to muscle test.

• Extend the arm that you use to write with out sideways at shoulder height.
• With the other hand, hold a crystal over a chakra or over the centre of your chest.
• Ask a friend to stand behind you and press down on your extended arm at the wrist, saying, "Resist."
• If the arm remains strong and firm, this is the right crystal for you. If the arm drops, try another crystal.

Purifying and Focusing Your Crystals

Purifying your crystal

As crystals hold the energetic charge of everyone who comes into contact with them and rapidly absorb emanations from their surroundings as well as your personal energies they need regular purifying. This is particularly so when they are being used for blocking or clearing. It is sensible to cleanse and re-energize a crystal every time it is used or at least weekly if in a grid. The method employed will depend on the type of crystal. Soft and friable crystals, for instance, and those that are attached to a base may be damaged by water or frost, and soft stones such as Halite or Selenite will dissolve. These are best purified by a 'dry' process such as brown rice or sun or moonlight, but sturdier crystals benefit from being placed under running water or in the sea.

Methods:

Running water

Hold your crystals under a running tap, or pour bottled

water over them, or place in them a stream or the ocean to draw off negative energy (use a bag to hold small crystals). You can also immerse appropriate crystals in a bowl of water into which a handful of sea salt or rock salt has been added. (Salt is best avoided if the crystal is layered or friable.) Dry the crystal carefully afterwards and place in the sun to re-energize or use a proprietary crystal essence.

Returning to the earth

You will need to dowse to establish the length of time a crystal needs to return to the earth in order to cleanse and recharge as the period will differ with each crystal. If you do not have a garden, a flowerpot filled with soil or sand can be used instead and is very handy for crystals that require a daily cleanse and regrounding. If you bury crystals to cleanse them, remember to mark the spot.

Rice or salt

Brown rice seems to have a special affinity with crystals that have been subjected to EMF or negative energy pollution, rapidly drawing it off. Salt – and Halite – also works but may be damaging to layered or friable crystals. Place your crystal in a bowl of brown rice or salt (unless layered or friable) and leave overnight for the negative energies to be absorbed – then compost or discard the rice. Do not eat. If using salt, brush it off carefully and make sure that it has been removed from any niches or cracks in the crystal as otherwise it will absorb water in the future and could cause splintering. Place the crystals in the sun or under the moon to re-energize if appropriate, or use a proprietary crystal essence (see Resources).

Smudging

Sage, sweetgrass or joss sticks are excellent for smudging as they quickly remove negative energies. Light the smudge stick and pass it over the crystal if it is large, or hold the crystal in your hand in the smoke if it is small. It is traditional to fan the smoke gently with a feather but this is not essential.

Visualizing light

Hold your crystal in your hands and visualize a column of bright white light coming down and covering the crystal, absorbing anything negative it may have picked up and restoring the pure energy once more. If you find visualization difficult, you can use the light of a candle. Crystals also respond well to being placed in sun or moonlight to cleanse and recharge.

Crystal clearing essences

A number of crystal and space clearing essences are available from essence suppliers, crystal shops and the Internet (see Resources). Personally I never move far without Petaltone Clear2Light, a crystal and space clearing essence and Petaltone Z14, an etheric clearer. You can either drop the essence directly on to the crystal, gently rubbing it over the crystal with your finger, or put a few drops into clean spring water in an atomiser or spray bottle and gently mist the crystal. Placing a couple of drops of Z14 on a crystal and leaving it in place for several months keeps the whole space energetically clean and protected.

If a grid has been buried, you can sprinkle a few drops of the essence into the general area and ask that it will cleanse and re-energize all the crystals in the grid. Petaltone Z14 is particularly helpful for grids as it clears fourteen layers of the etheric as well as the physical. Place a drop in the centre and invoke Archangel Michael to assist in clearing the area. Z14 can also be placed on a crystal such as Quartz or Selenite and left in situ to clear an area or to keep a crystal grid purified.

Re-energizing your crystal

Crystals can be placed on a Quartz cluster or on a large Carnelian to re-energize them. Or, you can use a proprietary crystal recharger (Petaltone and the Crystal Balance Company make excellent ones, see Resources) but the light of the sun is an excellent natural energizer. Red and yellow crystals particularly enjoy being placed in the sun, and white and pale-coloured crystals respond well to the full moon. (Be aware that sunlight focused through a crystal may be a fire hazard and delicate crystals will lose their colour quickly if left exposed to light.) Some brown crystals such as Smoky Quartz respond to being placed on or in the earth to recharge. If you bury a crystal, remember to mark its position clearly.

Focusing and activating your crystal

Crystals work best when their energy is harnessed and focused with intent towards the task at hand as this activates them. By taking the time to attune a crystal to your own unique frequency, you enhance its vibratory effect and amplify its healing power. Once your crystal has been purified and re-energized, sit quietly holding the crystal in your hands for a few minutes until you feel in tune with it. Picture it surrounded by light and love. State that the crystal is dedicated to the highest good of all who use it. Then state very clearly your intention for the crystal – that it will heal or protect you, for instance, or that it will transmute negative energy. If it is intended for a specific purpose, such as healing a particular condition or harmonizing space, state that also. Repeat the intention several times to anchor it into the crystal.

Deprogramming a crystal

There may be times when a crystal has been dedicated for one particular use but is no longer required for that purpose. This does not mean its usefulness is over. Far from it; it will undoubtedly have other work to do and another purpose to carry out. The crystal should be deprogrammed and rededicated before reuse.

As has been seen, crystals hold thoughts and intentions. Which means that if you have been gifted a crystal, whatever the giver envisioned or intended for you will be programmed into the crystal. Similarly, the crystal may be automatically imprinted with assumptions as to what that crystal does. The labels in a crystal shop or a description on the Internet is sufficient to do that. The deepest intention someone has may be unconscious and unacknowledged – and far from what they thought they were putting into a crystal. It is therefore sensible to thoroughly deprogramme a crystal and put your own intention into it before use unless you totally trust that the gifter of your crystal is attuned to your highest good.

To deprogramme a crystal

Hold the crystal in your hands for a few moments, thanking it for doing its work and for holding the intention and purpose it has had. Explain to the crystal that this part of its work is now over, and ask the crystal to dismantle the programme it has been carrying. See bright white light beaming into the crystal to help it to deprogramme, cleanse and recharge. Wash the crystal in Clear2Light and/or Z14 or other cleansing spray, or place it under running water. Put the crystal out into sunlight for a few hours or under the moon. The crystal may need a rest period to rebuild its energies before being rededicated to a new purpose.

If you are not visual: Cleanse the crystal with Clear2Light, place it under running water or into brown rice, and then into sun or moonlight. Then place the crystal on a Brandenberg Quartz and ask that it be returned to its original pure programme and purpose. Leave overnight. Then remove the crystal and allow it to rest before being rededicated.

How long should I use a crystal?

How long a crystal should be left in place depends on the use to which you are putting it. If it is for protection, you can wear it continuously as long as you cleanse it frequently. If it is to create safe space or for Feng Shui, it can also be left in situ for long periods and periodically cleansed. But if you are using it for healing purposes, then the time may vary between a few minutes to several hours or even days. Most crystals that are an integral part of a grid will remain in place for long periods of time but you can dowse to see whether they need cleansing, moving or replacing.

Crystal Essences

Crystal essences are an excellent way to use the healing power of crystals, and several crystals can be combined provided you dowse to check compatibility. The essence can be gently rubbed on the skin or sprayed into a room. Essences intended for adult use are usually added to a glass of water and sipped, or taken from a dropper bottle, or sprayed around the aura or environment. Crystal essences are made by transferring the subtle energies into water, which then stores the vibrations and transfers them to the physical or subtle bodies in exactly the same way that a homoeopathic essence works. The essence is bottled and a preservative – brandy, vodka or cider vinegar – added. If the essence is to be taken by those for whom alcohol is inappropriate, cider vinegar can be used as a preservative or the essence rubbed on the skin. A few drops of essence for spraying a room can be placed in a spray bottle of water and spritzed around a room. Add a teaspoon of vodka or white rum, or an essential oil, as a preservative if the essence is not to be used immediately. (See Resources for purpose-made highly effective essences.)

Caution: Some stones contain trace minerals that are potentially toxic (see the list in Contraindications) and essences from these stones need to be made by an indirect method that transfers the vibrations without transferring any of the potentially toxic material from the stone (see page 30). If in doubt, make the essence by the indirect method, which is also suitable for fragile or layered stones. Always wash your hands after handling one of these stones and use in a tumbled version wherever possible.

Making a crystal essence

You will need the appropriate crystal, which has been cleansed and purified (see pages 21–24), one or two clean glass bowls, spring water and a suitable bottle in which to keep the essence (coloured glass is preferable to clear as it preserves the vibrations better). Essences can be made by the direct or indirect method. The indirect method is suitable for friable, layered or clustered crystals as well as those that may have a degree of toxicity. Spring water should be used rather than tap water that has chlorine, fluoride and aluminium added to it. Water from a spring with healing properties is particularly effective.

Direct method

Place enough spring water in a glass bowl to just cover the crystal. Stand the bowl in sunlight for several hours. (If the bowl is left outside, cover with a glass lid or cling film to prevent insects falling into it.) If appropriate, the bowl can also be left overnight in moonlight.

Indirect method

If the crystal is potentially toxic or fragile (see Contraindications page 275) place the crystal in a small glass bowl and stand the bowl within a large bowl that has sufficient spring water to raise the level above the crystal in the inner bowl. Stand the bowl in sunlight for several hours. (If the bowl is left outside, cover with a glass lid or cling film.) If appropriate, the bowl can also be left overnight in moonlight.

Bottling and preserving

If the essence is not to be used within a day or two, top up with two-thirds brandy, vodka, white rum or cider vinegar to one-third essence, otherwise the essence will become musty. This makes a 'mother tincture' that can be further diluted. To make a small dosage bottle, add seven drops of the mother essence to a dosage bottle containing two-thirds brandy and one-third water. If a spray bottle is being made, add seven drops of mother essence to pure water if using immediately. For prolonged use, vodka or white rum makes a useful preservative as it has no smell.

Using a crystal essence

For short-term use, an essence can be sipped every few minutes or rubbed on the affected part. Hold the water in your mouth for a few moments. If a dropper bottle has been made, drop seven drops under your tongue at regular intervals until the symptoms or condition ceases. Essences can also be applied to the skin, either at the wrist or over the site of a problem, or added to bath water.

If a spray bottle is made, spray all around the aura or around the room. This is particularly effective for clearing negative energies, especially from the crystals themselves, or from a sickroom or an electromagnetically or emotionally stressed place.

Shungite water

Shungite water assists your body by removing anything harmful, such as bacteria and free radicals, and supporting your immune system. To become biologically active, water needs to have Shungite immersed in it for at least forty-eight hours. However, once the first batch is made, simply refill the filter jug every time you use some of the water so that it is constantly replenished. Wash the jug and the bag of Shungite at least once a week depending on how much water you have used (you can store the activated water and return it to the jug). Place the Shungite in the sun for a few hours to recharge or use a proprietary crystal recharging essence. Raw Shungite is more effective than the silvery tumbles, but, no matter how often the non-vitreous type of Shungite has been washed, it does tend to leave a very fine suspension of black particles in the water. This is harmless and part of the process.

Making the water

You will need:

2-litre filter jug

Fine mesh 2" bag of raw Shungite (10–100gm)

Place the mesh bag of Shungite in the base of the filter jug (if using tap water you can also use a commercial filter if the jug is provided with one).

Pour water into the jug until it is full.

Stand it aside for 48 hours.

Then top up the water each time it is used.

Cleanse the Shungite frequently under running water and re-energize in the sun.

Using Your Crystals

Many of the directory entries indicate a chakra link through which a condition can be healed or a chakra balanced, or you can dowse for or intuit this (see page 127 and *Crystal Prescriptions volume 4* for further information on the physiology of the chakras). Most crystals can be placed over clothing on the chakra, or over organs or the site of dis-ease, and left in place for 15–20 minutes or so. They can also be placed around the body, out in your aura or in your space or the environment to create energetic grids. Grids can be buried directly into the ground (choose dark, robust stones such as Black Tourmaline or Smoky Quartz and mark the spot so that the crystals can be cleansed regularly). Or, stones can be inserted into the ground to act as acupuncture needles. Crystals can also be taped in place, or worn for much longer periods for healing or prevention. They can be kept in a pocket, or permanently placed around your bed or a room or against a source of detrimental EMFs or environmental disturbance.

If your crystal has a point, place it point towards yourself, or point down if placed on your body, to draw in healing or re-energizing properties into your body.

Place it point out, or point down below your feet to draw off potentially toxic residues or emotional debris. If you are protecting your home, place the crystals point out to deflect or redirect negative energy and to harmonize the space. If you are drawing in beneficial energies, place the crystals point in. When you have placed the stones, close your eyes and breathe gently and evenly and allow yourself to relax and feel the energy of the crystal radiating out through your whole being or your environment. Hold the intention that the stones will work for you. (See also the effect of shape page 90).

You can also apply Crystal Essences (see pages 28–32). These essences convey crystal vibes to the body or the environment at a subtle level, repatterning your cells to optimum.

Healing challenge

Occasionally a crystal, especially when used for space clearing or toxicity release, will trigger a 'healing challenge' when the symptoms appear to get worse rather than better and flu-like symptoms may occur. This is an indication of physical, emotional or mental toxins leaving the body, or your environment, and is all part of the body holistically healing itself. It occurs particularly in stress-related or chronic conditions caused by environmental factors or psychic attack. It can be soothed and facilitated by crystals such as Smoky Elestial Quartz, Eye of the Storm, Spirit Quartz or Quantum Quattro and by drinking plenty of water (Shungite-infused water is ideal). If a healing challenge occurs use these stones for a few days until the symptoms dissipate and then return to the crystals you were using – having dowsed or intuited if they are still appropriate.

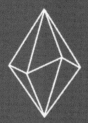

Part I
Space Clearing

Why clear your space?

Dictionary.com defines space as *"the unlimited or incalculably great three-dimensional realm or expanse in which all material objects are located and all events occur."* But I would beg to differ. Yes space is unlimited and incalculably great, but it is not three-dimensional. Space is multidimensional. It interweaves but goes far beyond our limited three-dimensional reality. Once we grasp this, so many things become apparent, and so many mysteries are explained.

Space is not dead either. It is full of constantly moving vibrations: detrimental or beneficial, discordant or harmonious. Space reflects what is around and within it. Chemical pollution, disturbed earth energies or geopathic stress may make itself felt. Everyone who passes through a space leaves an imprint of their energetic selves behind. You may even find that those who have passed on to another world pay a visit. To live in a state of well-being, you need to take energetic control and to cleanse, clear and contain your space bringing in the highest possible vibrations. The simplest and easiest technique of all is to dedicate and place crystals to keep your space clear. These may be single stones or grids that create an energetic net.

Space invasion

The human body emits low-level light, heat, and acoustical energy; has electrical and magnetic properties; and may also transduce energy that cannot be easily defined by physics and chemistry. All of these emissions are part of the human energy field, also called the biologic field, or biofield... We cannot isolate it or analyze it comprehensively. As John Muir wrote, "if we try to pick out any thing by itself, we find it hitched to every thing else in the universe" (Muir, 1911). For a field, this connection is especially true, given that, regardless of its source, it travels outwards to infinity, interacts with other fields by superposition, and interacts with matter along the way.

Dr Beverly Rubik in *Mosby's Complementary & Alternative Medicine*

There are subtle emanations and unseen vibrations everywhere. Thoughts and emotions leave an imprint, as does anyone around you. The past may remain energetically present. Electromagnetic frequencies and geopathic stress change the energetic ambience and can leave a space open to subtle invasion by less than welcome presences. You can easily recognize if there has been detrimental invasion of your living or working space. One or more of these symptoms will be present:

Space invasion – symptoms

- Feeling much better when away from the space
- Strong disinclination to be in your workplace or home (see page 75)
- Many arguments or small irritations
- Insomnia or panic attacks
- Excessive yawning or choking cough
- Feeling vaguely out of sorts and ill at ease
- Formerly clear crystals look murky
- A child or animal is disturbed
- Constant small infections and colds
- Light bulbs blow frequently
- Electrical apparatus malfunctions
- Unpleasant or unusual smells
- Cold patches
- The energy feels like walking through treacle

Similar symptoms may be produced by chemical toxicity from household chemicals or environmental or geopathic stress, and from mobile phone aerials, underground water, power lines, ley lines etc (see Environmental pollution page 292).

Space Healers

Atlantasite is an excellent stone to bury in the earth wherever there has been death and destruction as it clears and restructures the Earth's energy field to create a safe space. Blue, brown or white Aragonites are powerful earth healers that can be gridded around your house to keep the environment healthy and the neighbour vibes good. A beautiful pink Aragonite sphere fills your home with love and joy.

Creating safe space

The most difficult piece of the jig-saw is in trying to convince the people you live with that this area is your safe space and would they please respect it as such. Don't run through it with muddy shoes, don't play loud music when you want to use it, and if your co-habitees don't even share your sense of spirituality or your love of crystals, then ask them to at least respect your privacy when you want some time alone in your safe space.

www.hehishelo.co.uk/Creating-a-Safe-Space-for-Crystal-Work/B27.htm

The quality of a space very much depends upon those who occupy it. You cannot create a totally safe space if your emotions, motives and behaviour, or those of anyone who shares that space, are potentially toxic and not in alignment with higher energy principles. You need to clear yourself first and then your space. Bear in mind that 'as you think, so you are'. Staying safe means staying calm, positive, fearless and self-contained. Even if you share your space with someone whose vibes are not compatible, it is still possible to create a safe space within and around yourself. Carrying an Eye of the Storm (Judy's Jasper) helps you to be centred in a quiet, protected space no matter what is going on externally. A crystal visualization can also assist. It is particularly helpful when travelling or traversing difficult places or if there are disturbances going on around you. Remember to cleanse and dedicate the crystals you are using.

The Crystal Pyramid

- Where possible hold a crystal pyramid for this visualization and picture it expanding all around you. The floor sinks down as the walls move out.

- If you do not have a pyramid to hand, imagine that you are sitting in the middle of a crystal pyramid and the base is dropping as the walls expand out.

- The pyramid will have a floor as well as four sides that meet in an apex. Let it expand to be as large as necessary. (If you are protecting a room or a building, it should completely enclose this. If you are protecting yourself, it should go right around and beneath you.)

- When the pyramid is the right size, take your attention up to the apex. Picture a bright light coming in from the apex and shining all around the pyramid. Let this light sweep out the pyramid, transmuting any negative energies into positive ones. Then allow the light to heal and revitalize the space within the pyramid. State that higher helpers, guardians and mentors will be allowed into the pyramid but that everyone else and their subtle emanations will be barred unless you invite them in.

- Leaving the pyramid in place energetically, slowly bring your attention back into your body and be aware that you, the room or house are now protected by the pyramid. Take your attention down to your feet and re-earth yourself by allowing your grounding cord (see page 121) to pass through the base of the pyramid and into the earth (in emergencies withdraw the cable inside the pyramid).

- When you are ready, open your eyes and move around.

If you are non-visual: Use an actual crystal pyramid. Place it at the centre of your solar plexus and feel its protective glow *expanding to form a pyramid all around you. Keep the crystal pyramid where it will remind you of your safe space.*

If you have created an energetic crystal pyramid in a room, it can be helpful to physically place small appropriate crystals at each corner of the room to anchor the space and hold the energetic imprint so that the space remains clear and protected at all times.

Safe Space Grids

Layouts do not have to be large to be effective. Small crystals can be laid into protective and cleansing layouts such as the triangle, pentacle or the zigzag, or into energising layouts such as the spiral or sunburst. As some high vibration crystals can be expensive, placing one of these in the centre and adding clear Quartz points facing away from the centre amplifies and channels the energy outwards.

Judy Hall, *Earth Blessings*

Grids are the perfect way to protect your space. You can use as few as three stones or a plenitude. They can be laid in a small area, the energy generated will radiate out into the surrounding area; or a large space, to enclose and keep whatever is inside well protected. They can also be laid on maps or photographs of an area and will then work distantly at the area itself. Remember to cleanse your stones before laying them and to join up the lines with a crystal wand or the power of your own mind. If the line passes through a wall or other obstacle, pick up the line again on the other side. If grids are buried, mark the site so that you can cleanse the area regularly with Petaltone Clear2Light or Z14, or a similar clearing and recharging essence.

Triangulation

With just three stones you can clear and protect a large space. Large raw chunks are especially effective, particularly if they are to be laid around a building or the external environment (see page 51).

Triangulation grid

- Lay the first stone at the top point of the triangle.
- Lay the second stone to the bottom point, following the line down.
- Lay the third stone at the other point, following the line across.
- Join up the lines with a crystal wand or the power of your mind, remembering to return to the first point to complete the grid.

Star of David

The Star of David is an ancient symbol of protection. One triangle brings light into a space, the other clears out any negative vibes. Gridding your house with an upside down Rose Quartz or Selenite triangle to draw light in over an upward pointing Smoky Quartz or Black Tourmaline to clear negativity, for instance, creates a very safe and loving space. Use either tumbled stones, chunks of the raw stone or shaped pieces. This layout can be adapted to single rooms or to the whole area to be protected. It is not necessary to grid an upper storey as the energy grid that the stones create is multidimensional. Remember to cleanse and dedicate your stones before placing them, and frequently if they are left in place.

The Star of David grid

- With three Black Tourmaline, Smoky Quartz or other clearing stones, lay the first triangle beginning with the point at the top, moving down to the left to lay the second stone, and across to the right to lay the third. With your mind or a crystal wand, take the energetic line back up to the top.

- Feel the stones clearing the energy of the space, absorbing any potentially toxic, negative vibes.

- With three Rose Quartz, Selenite or other energizing stones, lay the first stone at the bottom of the second triangle, move up to the left to lay the second stone and across to the right to lay the third stone. Join the energetic line back to the bottom with your mind or a crystal wand.

- Feel the stones bringing in vibrant refreshing energy that spills out and fills the whole space.
- Leave the stones in place but remember to cleanse them weekly.

The Pentagram

The pentagram is another ancient symbol of protection that draws down light into matter. It is particularly useful for map or photograph work but will also clear and protect a house or environment. The topmost point represents Spirit and the other points the elements of air, earth, fire and water. If you wish to banish a ghost, poltergeist or traumatic memory from a space, lay an upside down pentagram. You can complete the pentagram by placing a circle of stones around it if this is appropriate.

The pentagram grid

- Lay a light-bringing stone such as Selenite, or other appropriate stone such as Aragonite for earth healing, on the top point.
- Follow the line down to a bottom point and lay a stone there.

- Follow the line up to a cross point and lay a stone there.
- Follow the line across to the other cross point and lay a stone there.
- Follow the line down to the other bottom point and lay a stone there.
- With a crystal wand or the power of your mind, follow the lines once again remembering to return to the top point to complete the grid.

(See also the sick building syndrome grids on page 58.)

Radiating energy layout

A sunburst layout fills a space with radiant energy – and can be combined with a semi-circle of protective energy to rebalance a space (see page 93). The lines radiate not only in a straight line but also in waves out from the centre creating a complex interplay of energies. Lay the central stone first and then place the crystals around it in a way that intuitively feels right, or dowse for placements. You can add several crystals to a line or just one at the end. Even a small sunburst will energetically fill a large space. Choose a large vibrant stone for the centre such as Citrine, Quartz, Carnelian or Jasper. Radiating grids are also suitable for placing on a map or photograph (see page 52).

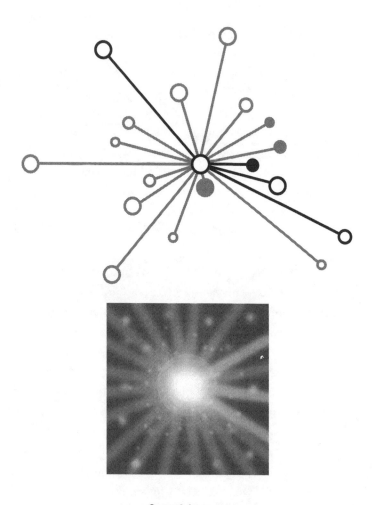

Spiral layout

Spirals are particularly useful for bringing seemingly 'dead space' back to life, restoring harmony. The layout cleanses and re-energizes, radiating energy into or out of a space. Depending on which way it is placed, a spiral draws energy down into the space or radiates it out depending on whether the crystal is laid at the end first or the centre. Dowse or use your intuition to check whether you should be using a clockwise or anticlockwise spiral and how many crystals are needed. When joining the crystals do not go back to the first crystal laid; spiral the energy out and away, or down into the centre.

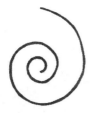

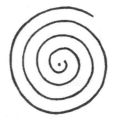

Clockwise spiral   Anticlockwise spiral

Outdoor layouts

If you are laying a crystal grid out of doors, remember to choose robust stones – clusters or layered stones will shatter if frost penetrates them and Selenite dissolves in rain. However, you can add a central stone such as Halite or Selenite soaked in Petaltone Z14 or an environmental essence to keep the grid energetically clear. This is particularly useful if the grid is to be buried in the ground as the Z14 effect lasts at least six months. The stone will eventually dissolve but that is part of the process.

- Cleanse your stones and state your intention.

- Open your palm chakras by briskly rubbing your hands together.
- Select your spot and grid shape by dowsing or use your intuition.
- Lay the grid out roughly to begin with.
- A long pole helps to establish that radiating lines are straight, or a ruler on a photograph can be used to check the alignment but you may have to allow for camera distortion.
- Adjust the stones if necessary.
- Join the lines of the grid as appropriate.
- If the grid is to be left in place for a long period, it can be buried in the ground but remember to mark the spot so that the crystals can be cleansed or include a central stone soaked in Petaltone Z14.

Map and photograph layouts

If you need to protect and space clear an area that, for whatever reason, is unsuitable for crystal placements or layouts, you can either take a photograph and lay the crystal grids on that, or lay them on a map. Place the crystals in exactly the same way that you would in the actual space and ask that the energy will be transferred to the site. Cleanse the crystals regularly.

Sick Building Syndrome

Sick building syndrome is a phenomenon whereby people experience a range of symptoms when in specific buildings. The symptoms are irritation of the eyes, nose, throat and skin, together with headache, lethargy, irritability and lack of concentration. Although present generally in the population, these symptoms are more prevalent in some buildings than in others, and disappear over hours or days when the afflicted person leaves the building concerned. The cause (or causes) are at present not clearly identified, but the syndrome can be discriminated from other building-related problems such as physical discomfort, infections and long-term cumulative chemical hazards such as asbestos and radon.

"Sick Building Syndrome", GJ Raw, Building Research Establishment Report

Sick building syndrome is not a myth. It is a reality as the report from the Building Research Establishment shows. Sick building syndrome occurs when a building literally makes you sick. This may vary from mild flu-like symptoms to extreme manifestations that create diseases such as cancer.[1] The environment within the building is unhealthy. It is characterised by static electricity and can be recognized by the high level of lethargy, vague 'unwellness' or excessive sick leave amongst employees in a business – or feeling better when you are not at home. Crystals can be used to harmonize the vibrations.

Contributing causes of sick building syndrome

- Excess static electricity
- Inappropriate construction materials such as asbestos
- Lack of natural light
- Fluorescent tubes
- Poor air circulation or ventilation
- High temperature
- Non-opening windows
- Low humidity
- Airborne particles and fungal spores
- Chemical pollutants from cleaning products
- Blown air heating systems
- Man-made fibres
- Paint
- Ozone from printers or copiers
- Proximity to high voltage power lines or electricity substations
- Underground power cables
- Smart meters
- WiFi and EMF pollution

- Excess positive ions

Sick building syndrome

A condition caused by a building with air pollution or inadequate ventilation, excess static electricity, electromagnetic smog, geopathic stress and the like. Symptoms, which include lack of concentration, headache, chest and skin problems, nausea, excessive fatigue, dizziness, usually disappear upon leaving the building and return on entering it again.

Symptoms of sick building syndrome

- Headache
- Clothes stick to you
- Excess static
- Dizziness
- Nausea
- Eye, nose or throat irritation
- Dry cough
- Dry or itching skin
- Shortness of breath
- Difficulty in concentrating
- Chronic fatigue
- Chemical sensitivity
- Sensitivity to odours
- Hoarseness

- Allergies
- Cold, flu-like symptoms
- Cancer
- Premature aging
- Increased incidence of asthma attacks
- Spirit invasion
- Personality changes

Excess static electricity

Excess static electricity literally gives you a shock. Surfaces and objects become charged. Sparks fly when there is static around. It may cause failure of sensitive electronics, dust clinging to surfaces, and objects apparently moving of their own volition. Touching door handles or other people can produce a sharp shock. Research by Peter Staheli suggests that static electricity may have an adverse effect on your health too as it interferes with the nervous system and bioelectrical processes in the body.[2] The energy requires grounding. Placing electrostatic crystals such as Jet, Amber or Tourmaline in a grid attracts the static to the crystal and grounds it. As does placing 'needles' of Smoky Quartz, Black Tourmaline and the like or a Halite (salt) lamp in the environment.

Static electricity or EMFs?

Staheli's research seems to suggest that it is the positive static electricity alongside high-tension power lines that may have contributed to the detrimental effects attributed to EMFs – although I would suggest, having researched EMFs extensively for *Crystal Prescriptions volume 3*, that it may well be a combination of the two creating too many positive ions.

> *High-tension power lines are essentially nothing else but man-made Chinooks or Foehns, which knowingly carry positive charged air that pesters people's nervous system. Chinook (wind) or Foehn, strong wind which blows on the lee side of a mountain range, such as the Alps (where it is known as foehn), when stable air is made to flow over the range by a large-scale pressure gradient. The air is dry and warm at the foot of the mountains; the wind undergoes further heating and drying as it descends the slopes. Such dry air masses are positive charged and feared by people whose nervous system is affected through it. Exactly the same characteristic as the positive ion clouds released by power lines. Also the suffering is the same.*
> http://www.royalrife.com/powerlines.html

Staheli's research has shown that a person lying in a bed that is insulated from Earth always takes on a positive charge. Similarly, people living close to power lines take on a positive electrical charge. If the bed is earthed with grounding crystals or surrounded with negative ionising crystals, the effect can be reversed.

Quick fix: Leave a Halite salt lamp burning or place a grid with appropriate crystals such as Black Tourmaline or Smoky Quartz around each corner of the bed.

Geopathic stress

A more serious form of sick building syndrome occurs when the building is on a geopathic stress line or suffers from severe EMF pollution. Looking back at the medical history of former occupants or employees can produce clues. If more than one of the previous occupants has had cancer, for instance, attention needs to be focused on the underlying energetics of the site (see *Crystal Prescriptions volume 3* for research and advanced protection measures). Placing an appropriate crystal between you and the source of the EMFs or moving a geopathic stress line with crystals will assist, as can the sick building layouts on page 59.

Geopathic stress

Earth and physiological stress created by subtle emanations and vibrational conflicts or disturbances from underground water, power lines, natural landscape features, negative earth energy and other subterranean events.

Layouts for sick building syndrome

Appropriate crystals (see A–Z Directory) can be placed at the corner of the building, or within a room or wherever a line of geopathic stress enters the building so that it is deflected. Join up the lines of a layout with a crystal wand or the power of your mind. Detrimental geopathic lines passing through a room may need to be blocked or moved (see *Crystal Prescriptions volume 3*). Choose appropriate crystals carefully. If the problem occurs because of excess static electricity, for instance, Amber and Tourmaline – both electrostatic crystals – could counteract it especially when balanced with Smoky Quartz or Selenite. Quartz having a stable piezoelectric 'pulse' restores energetic harmony.

The zigzag layout

The zigzag layout returns a sick building to a place of energetic peace. Place appropriate crystals as shown on the diagram below and cleanse them regularly. Crystals with points should all face in the same direction so that the energy is carried through and out of the building. If a wall intervenes, begin the zigzag again on the other side of the wall wherever possible. Placing detoxifying crystals such as Smoky Quartz or Shungite against a wall on one side and a light-bringing crystal such as Quartz or Selenite opposite works particularly well. If the syndrome is severe, however, and the symptoms return, you may need to ask for the assistance of an experienced dowser to move underlying geopathic stress lines. But sometimes moving house is the better option. Do bear in mind, however, that:

Should you find yourself in a chronically leaking boat,

energy devoted to changing vessels is likely to be more productive than energy devoted to patching leaks.
Warren Buffett

Sometimes moving house to be away from power or geopathic stress lines is the sensible option.

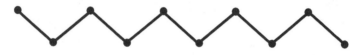

- Place a crystal on each point.

In a very large building, laying two zigzag grids, one on each side of the building, creates a complex, inter-weaving three-dimensional energy grid throughout the whole building. Place them in an inverted mirror fashion. That is, the detox crystals on the opposite side to that on which they were placed in the first zigzag so that they always remain against an external wall.

The energetic net effect of the double zigzag layout. This net is three-dimensional.

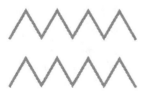

Negative Energy Lines and Geopathic Stress

Geopathic stress lines also contribute to sick building syndrome. But they can make your space feel very unsafe and have a detrimental effect on your health and well-being in any building.

As I explained in *Crystal Prescriptions volume 3,* in the same way that the physical body has a measurable bioenergetic sheath – the aura – around it, the Earth also has a subtle energy grid. This grid is created from, and interpenetrated by, a complex meridian matrix: intersecting energy lines, some geomagnetic, others electromagnetic, some telluric, others cosmic, that form a global grid through which powerful currents flow. These energies could be called the Earth's Qi or life force. They are like the blood, lymph and chemical messengers of the human physical body, cleansing and revitalizing all its organs and stimulating motion. The health and well-being of the Earth and all who reside in or on her body – the planet – depend on the healthy functioning of this field. These fields may not be in harmony, particularly where they intersect or interact with significant landscape features or man-made structures such as electricity pylons, buildings or quarries. If the grid is broken, disrupted or blocked in any way, especially by geopathic stress (GS) or the intrusive activities of humankind, the environment suffers. Anyone sensitive who is living there will feel out of sorts, disconnected and unnourished. Their physical body will also suffer.

Geopathic stress

Geopathic stress is also known as a 'black ley line' or adverse dragon line. It is created by subtle emanations and vibrational conflicts or disturbances from underground water, power lines, natural landscape features, negative earth energy and other subterranean events. GS can lead to physiological and psychological stress and dis-ease.

The effect of GS is found not only in the ground, it can radiate many feet into the air so someone living or working at the top of a thirty-three storey building could feel the effect as much as, or perhaps even more, than someone on the ground floor. Suitably placed crystals can harmonize, deflect or transmute GS, bringing conflicting energy currents back into harmony. The crystals can be placed at the actual intersection of the lines, especially where they pass through a home or workspace, or alongside fault lines, or on a map as the fields entrain no matter where in the world you may be.

Identifying a GS line

You can either work over a plan of the space to be checked out, or on a map, or in the space itself. Rods, pendulums or body dowsing are all suitable methods for identifying the lines. You will need to check out how wide a line is as well as the direction in which it moves and any other lines that may cross it. A crossing point benefits from a large Smoky Quartz or other harmonizing or blocking crystal, and lines can also be gridded – dowse for where to place crystals. Bear in mind that rooms often have several lines criss-crossing them and lines may bend. It's helpful to make a sketch as you work to keep track of them (see below).

To find a GS line in a room or out in the environment

If you are using a pendulum, ask it to show you the GS line and hold it in front of you as you very slowly move in a grid-like pattern up and then across and down until you have covered the whole area. Mark the points where the pendulum responds – remembering that lines are not always straight. Check that there are no other lines in the room by continuing the grid pattern, and working across the room in the other direction. You will probably find several lines. Mark the exact position as you go as otherwise you may have to check again.

If you are using rods, repeat the action above, watching for a response from the rods.

If you are finger dowsing, ask, "Please show me a GS line." Keep pulling your fingers until they hold together to indicate you have reached the line and open again when you have passed it.

If you are body dowsing, open your palm chakras and walk forwards, palms out. Or walk slowly placing your attention on your feet. Notice if your palms or feet tingle or go cold at certain spots or if it feels as though you are pushing against a wall of energy. Walk the same grid pattern so that you cover the whole room.

Note: If you are dowsing a bedroom and find GS lines, try to move your bed into a GS free space and neutralise the lines with crystals. (You may also need to move your mobile phone out of your bedroom as this is a major cause of EMF smog and disturbed sleep.)

To neutralise the lines

Place appropriate crystals at each end of the line where it enters a space and within that space wherever your dowsing suggests would be beneficial, especially at crossing points or where the lines enter a building and cross a bed.

In the example plan from *Crystal Prescriptions volume 3* shown below, there is a particularly strong line from a mobile phone mast (cell tower) passing through a bedroom (line A-B) and two other lines running from electricity poles and ground water cross it. Large Smoky

Quartz crystals were placed at the crossing points on the ground outside to deflect, harmonize and redirect the energies and replace them with beneficial vibes, together with large external crystals on the major line and other minor lines towards the property's boundary. A large Smoky Elestial Quartz was placed under the bed at the crossing point of the minor lines to transmute the effects. Black Tourmaline blockers were placed around the bed, on the lines and at the four corners of the room as the bed could not be repositioned. As the effect of the crystals kicked in, the placements were redowsed and crystals slowly removed until the optimum number was reached.

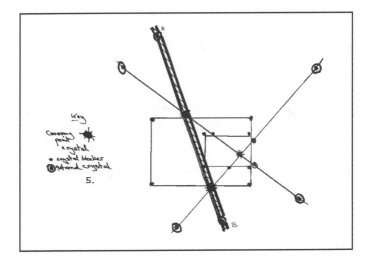

To find a GS line on a map or plan
If you are using a pendulum, ask it to show you the GS

line and hold it over the map or plan slowly moving it in a grid-like pattern up and then across and down until you have covered the whole plan or area. Mark the points where the pendulum responds (remember that lines are not always straight) and then join them up so that you see the line marked on the plan.

If you are using rods, repeat the action above, watching for a response from the rods.

If you are finger dowsing, keep pulling your fingers until they hold together to indicate you have reached the line and open again when you have passed it.

If you are body dowsing, open your palm chakras and use a forefinger to trace the grid-like pattern and notice if your finger tingles or goes cold at certain spots.

To neutralise the lines

Place your plan or map where it will not be disturbed, then place appropriate crystals at each end of the line or wherever your dowsing suggests would be beneficial. The map and the site will entrain. If possible also place crystals in the actual site.

Case History: Sick building syndrome and electrosensitivity

A client of mine had lived very happily in her flat for years. Although she had reached retirement age, she enjoyed excellent health. Until everything suddenly changed. She began to suffer from blinding headaches, debilitated memory, frequent colds, and visible trembling and shaking throughout her whole body that made her concerned that it was the onset of Parkinson's disease. However, when she looked at the situation, she was aware that the one change that had occurred was that the flats had been fitted with one of the new 'smart meters' to monitor and report on the use of electricity throughout the whole building. The smart meter, which covered all 20 flats, had been placed in the meter cupboard right opposite her front door.

Thinking that she would, however reluctantly, have to move she decided to try the Shungite remedy first. A very large raw chunk was placed above the meter cupboard on a high shelf where it would not be disturbed. Her symptoms receded. As soon as they began to return she cleansed the crystal thoroughly and put it out in the sun to recharge before replacing it. The symptoms disappeared again. Thereafter she cleansed and recharged the Shungite weekly. As an extra precaution, I suggested that she should grid the inside of her flat with a Black Tourmaline or Shungite grid in each corner. So far, her health has remained excellent.

Technological Vibrations and EMF Sensitivity

As we've seen, electromagnetic pollution (EMF smog) created by computers and other electrical and communication equipment has been shown to adversely affect physical and psychological health in sensitive people, as well as attracting the attentions of unwanted 'guests' (see *Crystal Prescriptions volume 3* for further details). If you are electrosensitive, you may find yourself prone to all or any of the following symptoms:

Electrosensitivity indications

- Severe energy depletion
- Immune deficiency
- Chemical sensitivity
- Chronic fatigue
- Loss of concentration
- Anxiety
- Allergies
- Inflammation
- Trembling and shaking
- Chronic infections or illnesses

- Negative subtle energy experiences

Even a few minutes under the influences of a sick building or EMF-soaked environment may drain the energy of someone who is electrosensitive. It creates insomnia and restless sleep. (You will find the full list of symptoms in *Crystal Prescriptions volume 3*.) If you are affected in this way:

Solutions

- Wear a Black Tourmaline or Shungite or other EMF protection crystal around your neck (see page 285).
- Stick a Black Tourmaline or Shungite plate to your mobile phone or tablet.
- Switch off your mobile phone or tablet at night and remove it from your bedroom.
- Do not use electric blankets or similar heating devices at night.
- Place Black Tourmaline, Shungite, Fluorite, Smoky Quartz, Lepidolite or Shungite on a computer, smart meter or other source of EMFs.
- Give thought to the type of lighting you use. Avoid fluorescent tubes, and blue spectrum light at night.

The anti-EMF grid

Grid your room with Black Tourmaline, Shungite or other EMF absorbing crystals, or place a large Black Tourmaline or Shungite between you and the source of the EMF smog. If the source is external, place crystals on the window ledges or in the corners of your room. A triangular grid works well as it radiates protective energy outwards as well as protecting the inner space. Place a crystal in each corner at the end of a wall and one midway along the facing wall.

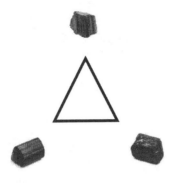

Triangular grid with crystals: Place a crystal on each point as shown.

Reversing a Chemically, Potentially Toxic, Environment

As we have seen, modern life generates potentially toxic energetic pollution that subtly affects your sense of ease and well-being. But it also generates chemical pollution. Chemical sensitivity invariably accompanies electrosensitivity and sick building syndrome. Crystals such as Shungite or Halite can assist in neutralising this pollution and may be used in various ways, one of the most effective being placing them between you and a source of pollution. But chemical pollution tends to be in the air that you breathe, so drink plenty of Shungite water to counteract this. Crystals can absorb and reverse the emanations into positive vibes that create healing for the environment. Halite salt lamps absorb chemicals from the atmosphere. Large quantities of Shungite can assist by absorbing toxicity in bodies of water and small quantities render your drinking water clean and wholesome (see Shungite water page 31). Remember to cleanse and recharge stones used for environmental pollution regularly. Choose your crystals from the A–Z Directory.

Environmental toxicity – symptoms

- Compromised immune system
- Insomnia or restless sleep
- Respiratory problems
- Chronic fatigue
- Skin conditions
- Behavioural or mood changes

Chemical pollution

Chemical pollution means the presence in our environment (e.g., air, water, soil) of chemicals (chemical pollutants) that are either not naturally present there or are found in amounts higher than their natural background values (amounts in which the chemicals are naturally present in a certain environment).

www.environmentalpollutioncenters.org/chemical/

Pesticides are just one of the chemicals we are exposed to from the environment; by-products of industry, plastics and synthetics we use daily, such as cosmetics and air fresheners, all make their way into our systems.

www.ec.europa.eu

The term chemical refers to the elemental composition of a material with a definite chemical structure. The mismanagement and overuse of these potentially lethal materials has degraded the environment throughout the twentieth century. Although the effects of chemicals on our planet have been most observable on a local scale, it is currently a complex international concern that lacks a pronounced solution. Without proper treatment and cooperation among actors, the ramifications of chemical misuse will permanently contaminate our planet.

www.environmentalgovernance.org

The sensible solution to chemical pollution is to closely monitor the chemicals that you yourself put into your environment. Avoid air fresheners and the like. Use natural fibres and organic products where possible. Certain natural chemicals are, however, actually potentially toxic so be careful when burning incense or using scented candles. Frankincense, for instance, is potentially toxic but its efficiency at supporting the removal of negative entities makes it acceptable for short-term use. Some crystals have potentially toxic minerals bound up within their chemical structure. Few of these minerals 'escape' when handling crystals, except when using raw lead-based crystals such as Galena (see Contraindications in the directory), but it is sensible to take precautions such as making essences by the indirect method and washing your hands after handling the crystals. Crystals such as Shungite, Halite or Hanksite assist in absorbing and restoring the balance where chemical pollution is present.

Harmonizing Your Workspace

You cannot function at maximum efficiency and maintain your vitality if you are operating in an atmosphere that is murky and cluttered. Creating a safe working environment is just as important at the subtle energetic level as it is at the physical. Computers and other electrical equipment create electromagnetic smog and stressed people pull the energy field down. Sick building syndrome (see page 53) is common and may affect well-being.

If you share an office or other working space, visualize a crystal pyramid before you arrive at work (see page 42). You can also keep a crystal 'paperweight' on your desk or regularly spray the area with a crystal cleansing or space clearing essence. A few drops of Petaltone Z14 on a crystal will keep the space energetically clear for several months but will need topping up when you cleanse the crystal. The most important measure you can take to keep the vibrations clear and beneficial is regular energetic cleansing.

If your work involves other people, especially if those other people are troubled, stressed or depressed, then you need to be particularly scrupulous about cleansing the space and protecting your energies. Many people unknowingly draw off negative vibes from their clients or colleagues. Cleansing and protecting your energies is vital if you work in the service, healing, care or therapy fields, but it is beneficial in other situations. (See the spleen chakra protection exercise on page 149.) If being around a particular person leaves you exhausted or depressed, you may have picked up some of their 'stuff' or unwittingly given them some of your energy. Your boundaries may be too diffuse and in need of a repair – Labradorite is excellent for this. If you find thoughts and memories of a particular person tugging at you, then it is likely that you have not completely disconnected from them. Check out where the connection is still holding – solar plexus, spleen or third eye – and use Green Aventurine, Banded Agate or other cord cutting crystal immediately. If you feel bullied or overwhelmed, you need both to protect yourself and to enhance your confidence. Do not wait until the end of the day to deal with these matters. Wear an appropriate crystal constantly and ensure that your base and earth star chakras are functioning well.

If your workplace is filled with constant disagreements and bickering, place Rose Quartz or other workplace harmonizer crystal on a windowsill or central part of the building so that the energy is radiated throughout. A large Blue Lace Agate facilitates communication and Sodalite assists with listening and paying attention to answers received.

A large piece of Smoky Quartz absorbs negative energies, as does Amber, but remember to cleanse the crystals regularly.

Space Harmonizer

Quartz in its various forms is one of the best space harmonizers there is. Place one centrally to harmonize the energies and keep the vibrations high.

Nightmare Neighbours

Every man has a certain sphere of discretion which he has a right to expect shall not be infringed by his neighbours. This right flows from the very nature of man.
William Godwin

We've all had them, the noisy neighbours who make life hell. But there is a simple solution. A large piece of Rose Quartz placed on the adjoining wall – or a square delineating your space if the noise comes from all around. It helps you to tune them out, and calms them down wonderfully. It is especially efficient placed around classrooms so that pupils settle into their work and don't disrupt the day. Children generally respond well to crystals of all types, but Rose Quartz or Shungite is particularly useful for lowering aggression and hyperactivity at home or at school.

If the problem is that the neighbourhood is violent or crime-ridden, Sardonyx is the answer. Grid it all around to keep your property safe from theft and intimidation. But be sure that your own integrity is squeaky clean in every way or it won't work.

If you have the worst kind of nightmare neighbours from hell and want them gone, use Kick Ass spray from the Crystal Balance Company (see page 354). It quickly moves such people out of your space. It works exceedingly well for visitors who have overstayed their welcome too. Simply spray around your space and off they go. (This combination crystal is now impossible to obtain so I sent one to Jeni Powell of the Crystal Balance Company to make an essence. It's just as effective as the actual crystal!)

If you ever feel guilty about protecting yourself from your neighbours, remember that true unconditional love sets sensible boundaries that protect from harm. Mutual respect is what is needed. If it's not there and communication has broken down, use a crystal:

A wholesome oblivion of one's neighbours is the beginning of wisdom.
Richard Le Gallienne

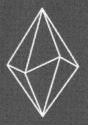

Part II
Crystal Feng Shui

Here Be Dragons

Over 4,000 years ago the Chinese recognized destructive earth vibrations that they called 'dragon lines' and warned against building houses on such stressful sites. The Chinese Emperor Kuang Yu (2205–2197 BCE) proclaimed, "No dwelling shall be built until the earth diviners have confirmed the intended building site to be free of earth demons"...

These hidden 'veins of the Dragon' carried 'vapours' (Qi or life force) and circulated, like the human bloodstream, removing impurities from the body of the Earth. However, they also deposited curative minerals (crystals) within it, and the currents were reflected in the Earth's atmosphere.

Judy Hall, *Crystal Prescriptions volume 3*

Feng Shui was created several thousand years ago by Chinese geomancers who recognized a need to rebalance noxious earth energies created in "the abode the Earth demons". In other words, earth energy lines that were detrimental to health and well-being. As I explained in *Crystal Prescriptions volume 3*:

This geomantic tradition continued and 3,000 years later Chen Su Xiao (d. 1332 CE) explained, "In the subterranean regions there are alternate layers of earth and rock and flowing spring waters. These strata rest upon thousands of vapours which are distributed in tens of thousands of branches, veins and threadlike openings." He said, "The body of the earth is like that of a human being. Ordinary people, not being able to see the veins and vessels which are disposed in order within the body of man, think that it is no more than a lump of solid flesh. Likewise, not being able to see the veins and vessels which are disposed in order under the ground, they think that the earth is just an homogenous mass."

However, Feng Shui does more than harmonize the environment. It also works for the home and workplace, and attracts abundance and good fortune into your life. Crystal Feng Shui smoothes out energetic 'whirlpools' and clears blockages to the smooth flow of energy by placing crystals in appropriate places. Highly polished 'auspicious crystals' including crystal balls reflect energy and turn it around corners where necessary, or slow it down if it is travelling too fast. Clusters and large points generate energy and so on. As the system includes colours, crystals can be placed to harmonize with hues of a particular area (see the bagua page 87). The crystals selected should be as large as possible and should be cleansed regularly.

Ammolite

Ammolite is called by Feng Shui masters the Seven Colour Prosperity Stone. An effective earth healing stone, they believe Ammolite stimulates the flow of *Qi*, life force, through the body or the earth. It is said that this stone is fortunate for anyone who comes in contact with it. Keep one in your home to bring wealth, health, vitality and happiness; and in business premises to promote beneficial business dealings. Wear it as jewellery, to impart 'charisma and sensuous beauty' to the wearer. Ammolite is available in different colours, use in accordance with the colours of the bagua and the effect required.

Traditional Feng Shui crystal colours

Red: growth and energy
Orange: creativity and increased libido
Green: wisdom, intellect, entrepreneurship
Yellow: wealth
Blue: peace and health
Purple: spiritual advancement

The Houses of Life

Some systems of Feng Shui are based on compass directions and include the five elements. Others utilise direction from the front door to create the bagua, the map of the house. The latter is the easier system to use when incorporating crystals. Placing a crystal in the relevant area of your home can radically transform the corresponding part of your life. Choose one to resonate with the colour, element or purpose of a specific placing. (See the directory page 295 for crystal suggestions.) When looking at the bagua, it is as well to bear in mind that each area covers a wide spectrum that may not be instantly identifiable from the title of the area – which may vary within different systems. In the bagua below, for instance, 'Love and Marriage' is in what I refer to as the relationship corner because it covers so much more than love and marriage. Partnerships of all kinds from business relationships to close friendships are enhanced by crystals placed in this area (see the case history on page 96). Similarly, 'Knowledge and Self-Cultivation', for me, translates into 'Inner Knowing and Self-Development'. This is the area in which to keep your spiritual growth books and crystals. 'Wealth and

Prosperity' is, from my perspective, the abundance corner that draws all good things into your life, not just money. Place your abundance crystals here.

Prosperity consciousness

Prosperity is a state of mind and a way of well-being. It is more than having money and possessions, although naturally these have their place. Prosperity consciousness is about feeling satisfied and secure with what you have, living an enriching and fulfilling life, sharing life's bounty, feeling gratitude and trusting that the universe provides appropriately for your needs... Abundance is all about appreciating and valuing yourself *exactly as you are right now*. Having an unshakeable sense of your own inner worth is one of the richest resources you have.

Judy Hall, *Crystal Prosperity*

WEALTH & PROSPERITY "Gratitude" REAR LEFT **Wood**	FAME & REPUTATION "Integrity" REAR MIDDLE **Fire**	LOVE & MARRIAGE "Receptivity" REAR RIGHT **Earth**
Blues, Purple, & Reds	Reds	Reds, Pinks, & Whites
HEALTH & FAMILY "Strength" MIDDLE LEFT **Wood**	CENTER **Earth**	CREATIVITY & CHILDREN "Joy" MIDDLE RIGHT **Metal**
Blues, & Greens	Yellow & Earth Tones	White & Pastels
KNOWLEDGE & SELF-CULTIVATION "Stillness" FRONT LEFT **Earth**	CAREER "Depth" FRONT MIDDLE **Water**	HELPFUL PEOPLE & TRAVEL "Synchronicity" FRONT LEFT **Metal**
Black, Blues, & Greens	Black & and Dark Tones	White, Grey & Black

Front door

Bagua using the front entrance to your home or the doorway to a room as a reference point.

The bagua can be applied to a single room or a whole house, an apartment or workspace. Colour or elemental correspondences heighten the effect. Golden Healer Quartz in the health area creates well-being for instance, but you could also use Petrified or Peanut Wood to resonate with the wood element of that area or Quantum

Quattro to fulfil the blue-green correspondence. Carnelian, Red Jasper or Fire Agate in the fame and reputation area would fulfil both the red and the fire element of that part of the bagua. Two Rose Quartz hearts placed in the relationship corner promote marital bliss and harmonize with the appropriate colour for that area. If a child tends to get overexcited and has trouble sleeping, a silvery polished Hematite in the area of children quickly calms them down. Hematite, being the mineral form of iron, belongs to the metal element that is appropriate to the bagua area for children. An earthy and earthing Eye of the Storm sphere in the centre of the house radiates an aura of calm throughout the whole space.

Services

The positioning of services in your home may need to be compensated for as they are unlikely to be movable. If your kitchen sink or toilet is placed in the wealth corner, for example, although you may attract money into the house it will continually be flushed away so you will never hold on to your money. Similarly, if the fame or career area is affected, your opportunities may go 'down the pan'. Placing a large Citrine geode, Shiva Shell or similar 'cave-like' crystal, a shape that conserves energy, on or near the cistern or close to the sink solves the problem.

Missing areas of the bagua

If your home does not fit neatly into the bagua, you can place crystals to delineate and 'fill in' missing areas. If the relationship corner is out in the garden or back yard, for instance, placing a large chunk of Rose Quartz where the missing corner would be completes the bagua. If the wealth corner is lacking and there is an appropriate covered area in which to place it, use a Citrine geode facing into the house to draw prosperity in and conserve it. (A geode or cluster will disintegrate if left out to weather.) Or, bury a large Citrine point with its point towards the house. Citrine has the ability to cleanse itself so can be a good choice of crystal for placing in the earth provided it is one solid piece. If there is no external space in which to place the crystal, pop it into the corner nearest to where that area would be.

The Effect of Crystal Shape

Crystals generate and store energy and the shape of a crystal, rather than its size, will determine how effectively energy is moved around a space.

Large points: Generate vibrant energy in the direction in which they are pointing. But even small points can be extremely effective. With the point facing towards you, they radiate energy to you. With the point away from you, they draw off or deflect negative energy, transmuting it as they do so. Use points wherever the energy needs a boost but avoid placing large points in a bedroom as they may cause insomnia. They can be positioned in dark or stagnant corners or where the energy is dense and heavy, but never face a point towards you in an area such as this as it will channel the energy straight at you. If energy needs anchoring or grounding, choose a large Smoky Quartz point. To deflect electromagnetic emissions, face a Smoky Quartz or Black Tourmaline towards the source.

Faceted: Faceted crystals reflect energy in myriad directions and can be in hung in windows or other spaces to break up a direct line of chi.

Geodes: Capture and hold vibrational energy, transforming it and releasing it slowly as required. Place them where energy needs to be gently reflected back to heal an area. They are particularly helpful in a bedroom or a child's room, or placed at an angle by the front door to reflect energy around the whole house.

Clusters: Radiate energy equally in all directions. Avoid placing a cluster near to your bed as the energy may be too strong. One in the centre of a space will fill it with revitalizing energy, however.

Spheres or balls: Radiate calm and slow down racing currents or chaotic energy, or conversely, speed up stagnant energy. They move energy smoothly around a space and absorb negativity. Balls generate light and harmony. The type of crystal has a specific effect. A large clear Quartz ball in the main living area neutralises negative emotions and prevents arguments, giving clarity on situations while a Smoky Quartz sphere grounds energy and defuses tension. A Rose Quartz sphere creates a gently soothing, nurturing energy in a child's room or love into a bedroom, while a Citrine ball alleviates money worries. An Eye of the Storm sphere in the centre of the house diffuses an aura of calm throughout the whole building.

Place your crystal sphere:

- Halfway down a small hallway that has many doors leading off.
- In a long, narrow and dark hallway at the end of the hallway to reflect light back.
- In the centre of a long unbroken wall or hallway – place the sphere as close to the centre as possible.
- On the sill of a window or mirror that is opposite the front door.
- Where a dagger-like energy current strikes a house from an approaching road, crossroads or a corner. Place the crystal in a front window or by the front door to divert the energy.
- Halfway down a set of rooms that open out of each other to slow the rapid energy flow.
- At the top of the stairs if these lead immediately up from the front door.
- In a dark corner or dead end to avoid a build-up of stagnant energy and to draw in light.
- If a road sweeps past a house rushing energy along with it, place a sphere near to or outside the front door or nearest corner (see page 94).
- By a cash register to attract good fortune to it.

Crystal Deflection

Careful positioning of an appropriate crystal deflects, speeds up or slows down energies whether in a room or outside a building.

Points are particularly useful if you need to deflect an energy that is coming directly towards you – place the crystal point out to deflect but be careful that it does not then channel the energy into an inappropriate area. If you need to draw energy in, place the crystal point in. You can also radiate energies more evenly throughout a space with a sphere. An appropriate layout assists the process.

The sunburst layout

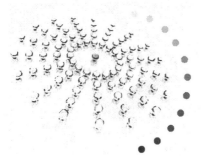

Sunburst with protective crescent layout

The protective Sunburst layout

A layout such as the sunburst-with-semi-circle will protect your space from detrimental energies coming from one side, and will radiate beneficial energy out to the other side. Create the semi-circle with dark coloured stones such as Black Tourmaline, Smoky Quartz point-out, or Shungite. Place a large Smoky or Clear Quartz point or sphere in the centre and create the radiating lines from Quartz, Herkimer Diamonds, Citrine, Selenite or other light-bringing crystals. If the crystals have points, face them outwards.

Diverting an energy arrow

If a road or other energy line heads directly towards your door, place a sphere or large crystal at the point of impact outside the front door to divert the arrow.

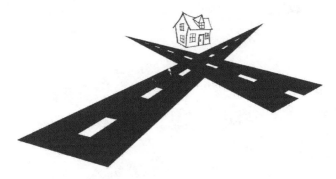

A house placed here would receive a dagger of fast moving energy from two directions where the roads intersect, which crystals placed outside the front of the house or just inside the front door could deflect. Energy could also rush past the house along the major road and an appropriate crystal to the side of the door would slow it down and harmonize it.

Feng Shui Case History

A writer lived in a house that had the bathroom in an extension added at the rear. It stuck out into the garden in the middle of the back wall, meaning that the wealth and relationship corners were missing when the house was placed on the bagua. To make matters worse, both the bathroom and the utility room below had WCs and plugholes located in the 'fame and reputation' area of the bagua. Although his books sold well, various other 'experts' in his field constantly trashed his reputation as their view conflicted with his: some going so far as to complain to the publishers about possibly injurious effects of the innovative content of his books. He was a prolific researcher and a thinker who was ahead of his time. There were two occasions when the publishers, always quick to pull books that have any taint of legal action, precipitately withdrew a book from the market. His agent did not back him or fight in his corner – the relationship corner of the house was missing and this encompasses relationships of all kinds. He had to provide convincing evidence and endorsements to back up his work – evidence which was already laid out in his books. Misrepresentation, distortions and jealousy were rife. There were many instances of "Joe Bloggs says… " going around and what would be quoted was the exact opposite of what he was actually saying.

As a consequence, his reputation and his income – remember that missing wealth corner – fluctuated wildly. I suggested he place a large Fire Agate, a red crystal, with a central 'cave' that resembled a geode on the back wall of both the bathroom and utility room. That would prevent his reputation being flushed down the pan. As geodes are not suitable for leaving outside for prolonged periods, he also placed a Citrine geode against the back wall where the missing wealth corner should be. A Quartz sphere in the career area of the house was then added as the stairs were opposite the front door and the energy rushed up the stairs and out through the bathroom. Placing the sphere at the foot of the stairs radiated the energy more equally throughout the whole house. To balance things out, he also placed a Rose Quartz against the missing relationship corner. Each corner was marked externally by a Flint to anchor the energy.

From that point on, things improved with great rapidity. His take on his field became the officially sanctioned interpretation seemingly overnight and his books sold increasingly well. He was in great demand on the lecture circuit. He found a new partner in the form of an agent who stood shoulder to shoulder with his clients. This agent negotiated much better deals than had previously been obtained. His career and reputation were firmly back on track. Thanks to crystals.

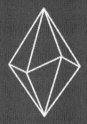

Part III
Psychic Protection

(Note: Some of the information in this section has been extracted and updated from Good Vibrations: Psychic Protection, Energy Enhancement, Space Clearing.*)*

The Need for Psychic Protection

You no doubt assume that you are well protected, but are you? Do you pick up other people's thoughts and feelings? Have you inadvertently upset someone? Are you particularly accident prone? Do you have a nagging pain under your left armpit? Do you constantly feel tired and listless? If so, you may be in need of a special kind of protection. Many people assume that, if they are working spiritually, they are automatically protected. But!
Judy Hall, *Good Vibrations*

When I wrote *Good Vibrations* the questions above were uppermost in my mind. While I did not want to worry readers unnecessarily and certainly didn't want to instil fear, I was very aware that there is an intrusive force that is silent, invisible, and yet which may be extremely powerful in its effect. Some people, especially those who dabble in the psychic realm or who open up spiritually without thinking of possible side effects, or who are electro- or chemically-sensitive, are particularly vulnerable. But anyone may inadvertently experience it at one time or another. This external force goes under many names: attachment, jealousy, resentment, aggression, ill wishing or, in its most virulent form, psychic attack. But there is an internal force that is just as deadly: self-loathing, hatred, anger, insecurity and so on. What we are dealing with is basically a projection of external *or internal* negative energy that is rarely recognized as an underlying source of dis-ease. Fortunately, crystals can protect you against this toxic tsunami and turn it around.

Psychic protection

Psychic self-protection creates a safe space in which to live, work and have your being. It is a protective barrier around the aura – the subtle energy field that surrounds you. Psychic protection acts as an impermeable barrier to other people's thoughts and feelings, especially if those are malevolent. Most people, at some time or another, have had the experience of having a thought pop into their head that doesn't belong. But, there are people who are constantly bombarded by other people's thoughts, and some have the misfortune to come under deliberate attack by someone who bears a grudge. Recreational drugs, meditation and yoga may also make you more sensitive to 'bad vibes', increasing your need for psychic protection.

Judy Hall, *Good Vibrations*

Signs that you may need psychic protection

- Certain people or places leave you feeling drained.
- Strong emotional currents constantly sweep through you.
- You are accident prone.
- Many small things have gone wrong recently.
- You lose things.
- You have nightmares and insomnia.
- You are anxious, nervy, on edge.
- You have invisible feelers out, testing the air around you.
- You are perpetually tired, listless, feeling hopeless.
- You feel invaded, somehow *not yourself.*
- You feel someone 'has it in' for you.
- You forget to detach yourself when contact with someone else has finished.
- You meddle or dabble in psychic things without being trained.
- You are psychic or have a sixth sense but don't know how to control this.
- You meditate without grounding yourself.
- You allow someone to have too much influence over you.
- You feel low if a friend is depressed or unhappy.
- You feel on edge if a friend is angry.

If you tick more than three or four of these, then you almost certainly need psychic protection.

Ask yourself:

Do I give away too much of my energy?

Do I detach myself after a contact is finished?

Have I taken on negative energy or emotion?

Am I allowing a person to have undue influence over me?

Am I taking enough time for myself?

See boundaries below.

You may also like to ask:

Do particular *places* affect you negatively?

Do certain *people* affect you adversely?

Do you get depleted when you travel on public transport?

Do you always sit in the same place and feel tired?

You'll find various solutions throughout this section.

Boundaries

If you have loose boundaries and are unable to say no to people or resist blandishments, psychic or otherwise, you could be in need of protection so:

- Are you able to say no?
- Do you take on too much for others?
- Do people come to you with their troubles?
- Do you feel overwhelmed by people's emotions or thoughts?

THE NEED FOR PSYCHIC PROTECTION

103

• Can you take 'me-time' without feeling guilty?

If you have loose boundaries see page 124 to strengthen and protect them.

Your body speaks your mind: check yourself out

Your body can quickly tell you if you are experiencing subtle energetic problems as it takes up a particular stance in response to a 'threat' even when you are not consciously aware of this. You will probably have instinctively folded your arms across your solar plexus, for example, or you may raise one shoulder as though to ward off a blow. Look at yourself in a full-length mirror and check out:

• Are your shoulders hunched?
• Is one shoulder raised as though to ward off a blow?
• Are your arms held tight across your chest?
• Are your hands clenched into fists?
• Do you have a defensive stance? Hands warding something off?
• Are you standing on tiptoe ready to run?
• Is your forehead puckered into a frown?
• Do your eyes dart about constantly monitoring your space?
• Is your neck tense and hunkered down into your shoulders?
• Are your shoulders tense?

- Or are you smiling, relaxed and standing tall, looking confident and serenely facing the world?

If you answer yes to all but the last point, then you are in fight or flight mode and need to relax and strengthen your energetic boundaries so that you feel safe within your body and your space. If you answer yes to the last question, you are well protected but may still need to be aware of techniques in case of a sudden breach of your energy field caused by walking into a negative environment, meeting a psychic vampire and so on.

Psychic energy drain signals
- Sudden loss of energy
- Chronic fatigue
- Nagging pain or tugging below left or right armpit
- Inability to sleep

The power of thought

The rice experiment is another famous Emoto demonstration of the power of negative thinking (and conversely, the power of positive thinking). Dr Emoto placed portions of cooked rice into two containers. On one container he wrote, "thank you" and on the other "you fool". He then instructed schoolchildren to say the labels

on the jars out loud everyday when they passed them by.
After 30 days, the rice in the container with positive
thoughts had barely changed, while the other was moldy
and rotten.

The Mind Unleashed[3]

When you have a negative thought either about yourself, or about someone else, it is unlikely that you stop to think of the effect it is having, either in the short or long term. A middle-aged woman, for instance, ranted on the phone to several friends about a young woman to whom her brother had just become engaged. In his fifties, he had appeared to be a confirmed bachelor, but he'd been bowled over and the relationship proceeded apace. The jealous sister, who had no relationship of her own, was convinced that the younger fiancée, who was not from the same country, was after his money and a visa and… and… The list was endless despite the fact that the young woman was well established in her own profession. The sister could not accept that they might be sharing a love that was mutual. The tirades continued for months. It was a prolonged psychic attack. When the marriage took place, the bride walked up the aisle suffering a nasty case of 'flu'. Which should perhaps have been called influence rather than influenza. Hardly surprising given the amount of animosity that had been directed her way and the powerful desire on the part of the sister to prevent the marriage from taking place. Had the bride been wearing Black Tourmaline or Shungite while the attack took place, she would most probably have skipped down the aisle in the best of health.

External psychic invasion

Psychic invasion comes from both the living and those who have passed on – especially those who have failed to move on in the spirit world. It may be deliberate, or inadvertent. Thoughts such as "I'll get back at you", "You'll suffer for this", "Why does she have all the luck?", or "I'll never forgive you" linger in the ether and surface long after the initial trigger. Jealousy, rage and resentment are particularly powerful psychic attackers, but someone's depression or black emotions can be equally debilitating. As can a parent who has passed on but is still trying, from the spirit world, to protect a child and especially when the parent does not approve of current actions. Former partners too may be reluctant to fully let go, and the connection remains in the chakras and auric field – whether the partner is in this or the next world. As this may be deeply unconscious, simply parting at a surface level may not be enough. Cord cutting may be needed (see page 181).

Internal psychic attack

Few people realise that their own toxic thoughts and emotions can be just as potent an attack on themselves. If you feel you are not good enough, not worthy and so on, you are constantly projecting your negativity on yourself. Other people may well pick up on it and reflect it back to you, but essentially you are attacking yourself. Time to stop!

The Right Kind of Protection

The key to good protection is to find exactly the right method for you and the situations you find yourself in. Practising techniques before you need them is sensible. But do bear in mind that what you believe in, you bring into being. If you feel safe, you will be. Positive thoughts and visualization (picturing things in your mind's eye) are powerful tools for protecting yourself, as is seeing the world as a benevolent place. Fortunately crystals can support you in taking a positive view, and protect you when the world is less than benign. At its simplest level, psychic protection is a crystal you wear, such as Black Tourmaline to block ill wishing, or a talisman you keep at your side to strengthen your energetic boundaries. It can be a bubble you inhabit (see the Amber Melt below). You need to take charge of your own thoughts and feelings and be fully grounded in your body: easily achieved with a few deep breaths and a grounding crystal.

> ## Protection is needed from:
>
> - Personal toxic thoughts and feelings.
> - Other people's toxic thoughts, intentions, ill wishing, jealousy and rage.
> - Environmental influences.
> - Soul loss, spirit attachment or thought forms.

We'll be looking at all these in this section, but before that familiarise yourself with the traps that leave you open to psychic invasion and in need of protection.

The stumbling blocks:

- Expectations and assumptions at an unconscious level.
- Toxic emotions held on to.
- Ingrained belief patterns and obsessive thoughts that go round and around the head.
- The language used to express what is going on in life.
- The lure of spells and incantations – chanting for wealth or asking the cosmos and so on may leave you wide open.
- People who have been inadvertently upset or who are jealous or resentful *whether or not they know you personally*.

Grounding

I'm starting this section with grounding because it is the single most effective thing you can do to protect yourself. Many people are vulnerable to invasion by negative energies simply because they do not have a strong enough connection to the planet. In other words they are ungrounded. If your boundaries are strong and you are rooted into the earth it acts like a firewall. Nothing detrimental can penetrate. But if your boundaries are diffuse or you are not connected to the planet, external energies may invade and drain. Ungroundedness occurs in people who are on a spiritual pathway, whether it be yoga, meditation or mindfulness, and who fail to keep contact between the earth and their physical body open. Having said that, if the Earth's own energies aren't sparkling clean where you are, it may be necessary to protect the earth star and Gaia gateway chakras with crystal light when you ground yourself to the centre of the Earth. If earth healing is needed beyond that given in the space clearing section of this book, check out *Earth Blessings* for in-depth assistance.

Symptoms of ungroundedness

- Mental confusion, unable to concentrate
- Inability to handle the everyday world
- Life and home are cluttered
- Eyes that show 'no one home'
- Spaced out, vague and unfocused
- Difficulty in motivating yourself
- Leaving everything to the last minute but not living in the moment
- Dizziness or 'woozy headed'
- Clumsiness and dyspraxia – you often bump into things
- Appearing to float several inches above the floor
- Sugar craving and a desire for junk food
- Constantly hungry but food doesn't satisfy
- Falling asleep while meditating
- Always running late
- Car or electrical equipment breaks down regularly
- Irritability without due cause
- Insomnia and restless sleep
- Unwanted out-of-body experiences
- Sense of looking down on yourself from above
- Body feels heavy and 'alien'
- Emotional and highly overreactive
- Constantly exhausted
- Great ideas or plans that never come to fruition
- Belching or breaking wind frequently
- Anxiety or unease with no apparent cause
- Displaying the same symptoms as someone you

were just with
- Mood changes suddenly when passing a stranger or entering a room
- Bank account is in the red

The Earth Connector Chakras

Four chakras are particularly important for keeping you anchored to the planet and your auric body protected so that you can ground higher dimensional energies and safely expand your consciousness. These chakras provide you with psychic protection.

The Gaia Gateway: anchoring Light to the planet

Location: About arm's length beneath your feet, below the earth star.

Qualities: A higher resonance of the earth star, this chakra anchors high frequency light into the physical body and the body of the Earth. Without this chakra high vibrational energy cannot be assimilated and grounded. It adjusts your electromagnetic frequency so that it remains in harmonic resonance with that of the planet *and* facilitates an uplift in your own personal resonance. This chakra connects you to the soul and spirit of the planet, Gaia, and to Mother Earth herself. When your Gaia gateway is open and functioning at optimum, you are aware of being a part of a sacred whole, part of the energy system of the Earth and, at the same time, All That Is. When balanced and open, this chakra helps you to protect yourself from entity attachment and lower energies.

Connective correspondence: Stellar gateway chakra.

Overactive/blown/spin too fast: When this chakra is blown it leads to extreme sensitivity to earth changes and to geopathic and electromagnetic stress. Being in incarnation, and especially being in a physical body, is challenging and there is no ability to remain stable during periods of energetic uplift.

Underactive/blocked/spin too slow: When this chakra is blocked there is an inability to ground and connect with higher energies. Disconnection from the Earth as a sacred, living being may lead to greed and over-utilisation of the planet's resources and consequent disregard for others who share the planet.

The Earth Star: everyday reality and groundedness

Location: About a foot beneath the feet.

Qualities: The earth star chakra connects you to the Earth's core as well as its electromagnetic fields and energy meridians. This chakra helps you to bring things into concrete form, grounding and anchoring new frequencies and actualising your plans and dreams. It is a place of safety and regeneration. Without it, you will have only a toehold in incarnation and be physically and psychologically ungrounded. With it, you have a stable, calm and strong centre from which to handle the vicissitudes of life and its pleasures with equal composure. When the chakra is functioning at optimum you have a natural electrical circuit providing a physical and spiritual energy boost. The sciatic nerve, the longest nerve in the body, runs from the heel of the foot up the legs to the hips and then across and into the spine. Passing up the spine it connects your brain to the vibrations of the Earth. It also connects your earth star chakra with the knee chakras and those chakras to the base so that you are fully grounded and connected to the physical dimension of being.

Connective correspondence: The soul star chakra.

Overactive/blown/spin too fast: If your earth star is blown you will lack grounding and have no connection to the planet or awareness of being part of a greater overall system. Or, paradoxically, you may be overly concerned for the planet and not give enough attention to your own body. An out of balance earth star easily picks up adverse environmental factors such as geopathic stress and toxic pollutants. It is highly sensitive to electromagnetic energy as it governs the electrical systems of the body and is your connection to the planet through the soles of your feet with their many nerve endings and minor chakras.

Underactive/blocked/spin too slow: Earth star blockages or disruptions lead to discomfort in your physical body, a sense of not belonging on the planet. With little body awareness, there are feelings of helplessness and ungroundedness accompanied by an inability to function practically in the world. You will be unable to assimilate higher dimensional energies.

The Knee Chakras: flexibility, balance and willpower

Location: Behind and through the knees, like a flat disc on which the body rests.

Qualities: When working well the knee chakras ensure you are flexible and able to adapt to changing circumstances. Literally able to 'go with the flow' and yet having perseverance when required. You are able to use your willpower to manifest a desired outcome. All the major energy meridians of the body pass through the knees as well as the longest nerve in the body, the sciatic. These chakras ensure that you have the ability to nurture and support yourself and manifest what you need on a day-to-day basis. When the knee chakras are balanced, you set realistic goals and outcomes, and let go when appropriate.

Not only can the knee chakras be blocked or too open, but they may also suffer a left-right imbalance, so check out each chakra and harmonize them with appropriate crystals. Generally speaking (but check it out for yourself), the left knee represents the feminine, yin aspect, that is receptive, emotional and intuitive. It is connected to the intuitive right hemisphere of the brain. The right knee represents the male, yang, aspect that is factual, practical, managerial and outgoing. It is connected to the rational left side of the brain.

Connective correspondence: The earth star, base, sacral and dantien.

Overactive/blown/spin too fast: When this chakra is blown, you will be overly impulsive and act before thinking, aggressively pushing through obstacles. You will be unable to negotiate or compromise. A blown knee chakra constantly meets problems with authority, authority figures and bureaucracy. There is a need to be in control. Arrogant superiority is common. This is the person who thinks he, or she, 'knows best' and so demands subservience from others. Control-freakery is common.

Underactive/blocked/spin too slow: Chronic fear and feelings of inferiority, and consequent subservience result from blocked knee chakras. Unhealthy dependent and controlling relationships including 'codependency', or difficulties in intimacy and closeness are common. You will be constantly challenged by others. The soul is not grounded into the earth plane, or practical everyday reality, and so feels empty.

The Dantien: powerfulness, energy regulation

Location: Two–three fingerbreadths (3–5 cm) below the navel, rotating on top of the sacral chakra.

Qualities: The dantien is your centre of gravity. It is an energy vortex and storage vault rather than a chakra per se. An adjunct to the sacral chakra and the point of balance for the physical body, the dantien is where Qi or prana, life force, is stored and your body earthed. Acting like a reservoir, this is your core energy source. It is a place of inner strength, stability and balance. This chakra is where you become centred around your inner core. When you are connected to your core, you not only have more physical energy as you are not affected by life's ups and downs, but you are also more emotionally stable and better able to resist stress. You are not easily thrown off balance. Nor are you open to manipulation by other people. When the dantien is full, you have inner resources to draw on. You are literally power-full. When it is functioning well you are energized and power-full, stable and well grounded.

Connective correspondence: Higher resonance of the sacral chakra.

Overactive/blown/spin too fast: If the dantien is too open, energy constantly drains out and chronic lethargy results. Many projects will be started but you will have no stamina or perseverance to complete them. You will also be easily pushed around or manipulated by other people, despite feeling that you are in control.

Underactive/blocked/spin too slow: Qi (life force) cannot circulate efficiently and is not replenished. The autoimmune system cannot function, with resultant dis-ease. Ideas cannot be put into practice and creativity is blocked.

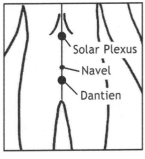

Solutions to Ungroundedness

In addition to keeping the earth connector chakras cleansed and well-balanced, grounding crystals (see A–Z Directory) in your pockets or around your bed can assist in anchoring you to the Earth. Belly breathing also helps to ground you to the planet and the grounding cord meditation practised daily until it becomes second nature is extremely effective. It doesn't restrict you to the planet; indeed it can make journeys to other dimensions much more powerful because it enables you to bring the information back into the physical plane of awareness.

Belly breathing

Before you begin, place a grounding crystal such as Flint or Hematite at your feet.

Hold a belly breathing crystal loosely over your dantien (just below your navel). Stand or sit with your feet firmly on the floor and your knees relaxed. Letting your shoulders hang low and loose, take a long, slow breath. Deliberately push out your ribs and belly and pull the breath deep into the base of your lungs towards the crystal. Feel your ribs expanding outwards at the back and sides, and your back and solar plexus opening up.

Breathe in for a count of four (increase the count with practice), hold the breath for a count of two, and exhale slowly pulling your belly and ribs in to expel all the air for a count of ten. Press your ribs in with your arms if necessary. Rest a moment and take another breath. Repeat eight times more (stop immediately if you feel light-headed and take your attention down to your feet, putting your feet on the earthing crystal or bouncing your feet firmly on the earth). Return to your normal breathing pattern but remember to pull the air deep down into your lungs.

The grounding cord

- Stand with your feet slightly apart, well balanced on your knees and hips. Feet flat on the floor. Place a Flint or other grounding stone at your feet and hold Poppy Jasper or other suitable stone over your dantien.
- Picture the earth star chakra about a foot beneath your feet opening like the petals of a water lily.
- Feel two roots growing from the soles of your feet down to meet at the earth star.
- The two roots twine together and pass down through the earth star and the Gaia gateway, going deep into the Earth. They pass through the outer mantle, down past the solid crust and deep into the molten magma.
- When the entwined roots have passed through the magma, they reach the big iron crystal ball at the

centre of the planet.

- The roots hook themselves around this ball, holding you firmly in incarnation and helping you to be grounded in incarnation.
- Energy and protection can flow up this root to keep you energized and safe.
- Allow the roots to pass up from the earth star through your feet, up your legs and the knee chakras and into your hips. At your hips the roots move across to meet in the base chakra, expanding from there to the sacral and the dantien. The energy that flows up from the centre of the Earth can be stored just below your navel in the dantien.

If you are non-visual: Massage the centre of the soles of your feet until they tingle and then place them firmly on the earth with a grounding crystal between them. Sense your grounding root growing from there and then up to a dantien crystal that you hold just below your navel.

Note: Whenever you are in an area of seriously disturbed earth energy, protect your earth star chakra by visualizing a large protective crystal all around it. The root will still be able to pass down to the centre of the Earth to bring powerful energy to support you, and the crystal will help to transmute and stabilize the negative energy.

If your boundaries are too diffuse:
Complete the grounding cord exercise first and then:

- Picture a large crystal bubble growing from the earth star chakra to enclose you, going all around your body and up to the soul star chakra above your head at arm's length from your body. Then picture another crystal bubble going from the Gaia gateway to the stellar gateway chakra. Wear a Labradorite, Healer's Gold or other boundary or firewall crystal pendant at all times (see also page 268) or carry Boji Stones in your pockets.

Boundaries: Instant protection

I make no apology for once again including one of my favourite protection practices. I find it invaluable for strengthening weak boundaries and providing emergency protection. A tiny piece of *The Amber Melt* is all you need:

The Amber Melt

- Close your eyes and breathe deeply, grounding yourself on the Earth.
- Breathe gently and hold a piece of Amber over your head (or place it at your head if you're lying down).

- Put all your attention into the crystal.
- Feel the Amber slowly melting and trickling like honey all around your auric field until it completely coats it, meeting under your feet.
- Feel how safe it is within your Amber cloak, how secure, and how you can easily find your centre and connection with the Earth within this beautiful crystal.
- Allow the crystal to draw off and transmute any negative energy or fearful emotions, de-stressing you and filling you with positive self-regard and

inner peace.

- Feel how, from the top of your head down into your heart, and on down to the earth beneath your feet, you have a central core of deep peace you can lean and rely on.
- When you're ready, withdraw your attention from the crystal but leave your bubble in place so that when you return your attention into the room you'll still have that core of inner peace.
- Stamp your foot to ground yourself back into the everyday once more.

This also works well using Polychrome Jasper or Eye of the Storm (Judy's Jasper). The different colours naturally present in the Jasper weave strands of protection all around your auric field. Wear the stones constantly to give you continued protection.

Firewalls

If you come under ill wishing or psychic attack, then what you require is a 'firewall' all around your aura rather than an interface. An interface allows an interchange of energy; a firewall does not. Choose your firewall crystals from the A–Z Directory. Ones with a strong metal content such as Tantalite are excellent but Fire Agate can be very potent.

Psychic Protection and
the Chakras

Before we look at specific protection methods, we need to look at the role the chakras play. How open or closed your chakras are has a powerful influence on your need for protection in specific areas of life – and also your openness to other people. These vortexes mediate the flow of energy between the physical and subtle energy bodies (see page 159 and *Crystal Prescriptions volume 4*, chakras and kundalini). They also create a boundary, a kind of energetic interface, between you, your aura and the outside world. If a chakra is spinning wildly out of control, in other words is too open, energy may whirl way out and be vampirised – 'fed upon' – by needy people. This may occur with those in a physical body, who may do it unconsciously, or discarnate souls who still crave the experiences of Earth. Conversely, if a chakra is blocked and spinning sluggishly, it can entrap energy or thoughts belonging to other people – 'alien energy' – within it, polluting your entire energy system.

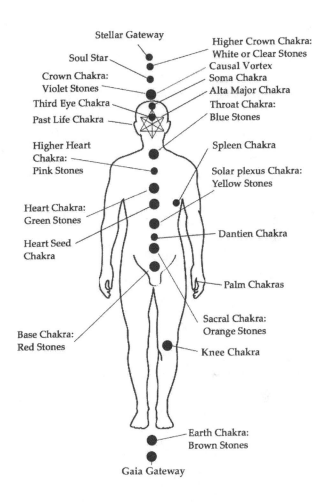

Stellar Gateway

Soul Star

Crown Chakra:
Violet Stones

Third Eye Chakra

Past Life Chakra

Higher Heart
Chakra:
Pink Stones

Heart Chakra:
Green Stones

Heart Seed
Chakra

Base Chakra:
Red Stones

Higher Crown Chakra:
White or Clear Stones
Causal Vortex
Soma Chakra
Alta Major Chakra
Throat Chakra:
Blue Stones

Spleen Chakra

Solar plexus Chakra:
Yellow Stones

Dantien Chakra

Palm Chakras

Sacral Chakra:
Orange Stones

Knee Chakra

Earth Chakra:
Brown Stones

Gaia Gateway

The chakras, a quick overview:

Gaia gateway: Connection to the planet, the collective
and the ancestors

Positive qualities: Concerned for the planet, able to
recognize collective and ancestral traits and heal these

where necessary.

Negative qualities: Too open to collective or ancestral influence, dependent: unable to stand on own two feet.

Vulnerabilities: Peer and transgenerational pressure, greed.

Earth star: Groundedness and ability to handle the everyday world

Positive qualities: Well grounded, practical, operates well in everyday reality.

Negative qualities: Ungrounded, impractical, picks up negativity.

Vulnerability: Negative earth energies and environmental disturbance.

Base: Basic security, survival instincts

Positive qualities: Good sense of your own power, independent.

Negative qualities: Vengeful, impotent, hyperactive, fearful, envious.

Vulnerability: Gives away power to others.

Knees: Connection to everyday world

Positive qualities: Well grounded, centred, handles everyday reality well.

Negative qualities: 'Air-head', disconnected from reality, unable to make decisions.

Vulnerability: Unable to distinguish reality from fantasy.

Sacral: Creativity, procreation

Positive qualities: Fertility, courage, assertion, acceptance of sexuality.

Negative qualities: Low self-esteem, inferiority, infertility, sluggish.

Vulnerability: Too much reliance on others.

Dantien: Power utilisation

Positive qualities: Empowered, able to handle power well, vital and full of well-being.

Negative qualities: Disempowered, arrogant, chronically exhausted.

Vulnerability: Susceptible to powerful people's influence.

Solar plexus: Emotional connection

Positive qualities: Good energy assimilation, empathic.

Negative qualities: Overly emotional or cold, emotional baggage.

Vulnerability: Takes on other people's feelings. Prone to energy leeching.

Spleen: Energy utilisation

Positive qualities: Self-contained, powerful.

Negative qualities: Exhausted and manipulated.

Vulnerability: Open to energy leeching.

Heart seed: Soul remembrance

Positive qualities: Remembers reason for incarnation, connection to divine plan, tools available to manifest potential.

Negative qualities: Rootless, purposeless, lost.
Vulnerability: Lack of sense of self.

Heart: Love and relationships
Positive qualities: Loving, generous, compassionate, accepting, empathetic.
Negative qualities: Heartless, disconnected from feelings, jealous, insecure.
Vulnerability: Tied to past contracts, desperate for love.

Higher heart: Unconditional love and immune system
Positive qualities: Forgiving, accepting, spiritually connected.
Negative qualities: Spiritually disconnected, grieving, needy.
Vulnerability: Becomes a doormat to abuse masquerading as 'love'.

Throat: Communication and self-expression
Positive qualities: Able to speak your own truth, receptive.
Negative qualities: Unable to verbalise thoughts/feelings, dogmatic.
Vulnerability: Liable to create thought forms through thoughtless words.

Third eye: Intuition and mental connection
Positive qualities: Intuitive, perceptive, visionary.
Negative qualities: Spaced-out, fearful, attached to past.
Vulnerability: Open to undue influence and thought form

attachment.

Soma: Spiritual connection
Positive qualities: Spiritually aware and fully conscious.
Negative qualities: Cut off from spiritual nourishment and connection.
Vulnerability: Not connected to the physical body.

Past life: Previous life experience
Positive qualities: Wisdom skills, instinctive knowing.
Negative qualities: Emotional baggage and unfinished business.
Vulnerability: Tries to live out past their sell-by-date soul intentions and contracts.

Crown: Spiritual connection
Positive qualities: Mystical, humanitarian, giving service.
Negative qualities: Overly imaginative, arrogant, uses power to control others.
Vulnerability: Open to invasion.

Soul star: Spiritual enlightenment/illumination
Positive qualities: Ultimate soul connection, objective perspective on past.
Negative qualities: Spiritual arrogance, soul fragmentation, rescues not empowers.
Vulnerability: Messiah-complex.

Stellar gateway: Cosmic doorway to other worlds

Positive qualities: Communication with enlightened beings.

Negative qualities: Disintegration, no boundaries.

Vulnerability: Open to cosmic disinformation.

Causal vortex: Ancestral and karmic memories

Positive qualities: Following own path, 'junk DNA' (see *Crystal Prescriptions volume 6*) is working effectively.

Negative qualities: Toeing the ancestral line, 'junk DNA' is polluted.

Vulnerability: Transgenerational expectations and pressures.

Alta major: The subtle hormonal and energy systems of the body

Positive qualities: Physical and subtle bodies are in harmony and functioning well.

Negative qualities: Physical and subtle bodies are out of alignment and unable to protect against invasion.

Vulnerability: Unacknowledged personal thoughts and emotions create dis-ease.

See also page 135.

Chakra Attachments

Chakras may be blocked by an attaching spirit, thought, emotion or belief. It's not only discarnate spirits that may attach here. The living may affect you too. Anyone you have ever had sex with could have left some of their energy field or a 'hook' in your lower chakras, for instance, but strong thoughts of lust can lodge there even if there has been no physical contact. Thought is a very powerful thing and thought forms or strong belief systems can easily affect the chakras especially around the head, throat and base (see page 156). It is also common to find that miscarriages or stillbirths have left behind some of the energy of the soul who could have been born, especially if there is an unfulfilled soul contract operating behind the scenes. You may find emotional attachment hooks in the spleen, sacral and solar plexus chakras; thought forms in the third eye and soma; ancestral hooks in virtually all the chakras but especially the causal vortex, alta major and base chakras.

Soul contract

A promise or agreement made in a previous life or the interlife. Such promises usually involve looking after someone or performing some kind of service to assist their soul plan.

An integrated defence system

The chakras form part of an integrated defence system along with your subtle body and your endocrine system. Crystals create an appropriate interaction in cooperation with the relevant chakras and the auric field (see the A–Z Directory). Labradorite and Healer's Gold are excellent crystals for creating a psychic interface, for instance. A point where your energies meet those of someone with whom empathy is required. You can sense what they are going through without being overwhelmed by 'their stuff'. Putting one of these crystals around your neck so that it is level with the higher heart chakra (see page 303) allows you to have insights while maintaining an appropriate boundary around your aura.

Ill wishing and psychic attack occur at a mental level and need to be stopped in their tracks, so Black Tourmaline or Shungite are appropriate crystals to place over the higher heart and mental chakras to not only block but also to absorb the energy. Bronzite, often sold as a protection against 'curses', does not absorb. It simply bounces the energy back and forth, exacerbating it in the process. Vampirisation of energy occurs at a more emotional level and can be blocked at the spleen or solar plexus chakras with Green Aventurine, Green Jade and similar stones (see page 349). This seals the energy portal through which energy is leaking and strengthens the auric field.

Chakra attachments

Gaia gateway (below the earth star): Planetary connection

Attachments: Cosmic, racial and collective spirits, often those who were dispossessed of their lands or ethnically cleansed.

Earth star (below the feet): Material connection

Attachments: Spirits of place, stuck spirits. Those who wish you to walk in their footsteps. If it is permanently open, you can easily pick up negative energies from the ground or pick up 'spirits of place', either as attachments or as communication of events that have taken place.

Knee: Flexibility, balance and willpower

Attachments: Those who want you to walk in their footsteps – ancestral spirits or past life personas that have a different agenda to your present soul intention.

Palm: Energy manifestation, transmutation and utilisation

Attachments: Energy drawn from anyone you've shaken hands with or touched in any way, also negative energy from objects or the environment. Anything you wished to hold on to in a previous life.

Base and sacral: Creativity

Attachments: Ancestral figures, previous partners, children, anyone you've ever had sex with, needy people, thought forms, unborn children and parents. Previous partners or significant others leave their imprint in these chakras and may continue to influence through the association. Sex addiction way back in the family may overstimulate these chakras and manifest in the present.

Dantien: Power utilisation

Attachments: Energy leeches, control freaks, disembodied spirits seeking energy to remanifest or move on, past life personas.

Solar plexus: Emotions

Attachments: People with whom you have had an emotional entanglement in the past whenever that may have been. Ancestral spirits, relatives, needy people. Invasion and energy leeching take place through this chakra. A 'stuck-open' solar plexus means you take on other people's feelings easily. You may well receive intuitions through your solar plexus as you unconsciously read other people's emotions.

Spleen (under left arm): Energy

Attachments: Psychic vampires, needy people, ex-partners. Psychic vampires can leech your energy, as can past partners, children or parents, and hooks here are common.

Heart seed (base of breastbone): Soul remembrance

Attachments: Parts of your soul left in other lives or dimensions. If you have left parts of yourself at past life deaths or traumatic or deeply emotional experiences, then these parts may be attached and trying to influence you to complete unfinished business.

Higher Heart (above the heart): Unconditional love

Attachments: Guides, gurus or masters, mentors. Mentors, masters and gurus open the higher heart chakra, and in so doing tie you to them and not all masters or gurus have clean energy or the best of intentions.

Throat (over throat): Communication

Attachments: Teachers, mentors, gurus, thought forms. A blocked throat chakra results in difficulty in communication – especially in not being able to speak your truth. Problems may arise from your own unvoiced intuitions and the dogmatic nature of a blocked throat chakra can leave you closed to intuitive solutions.

Third Eye (slightly above and between the eyebrows): Intuition

Attachments: Thought forms, ancestors or relatives, lost souls. If the chakra is blocked, then you cannot visualize or receive intuitions. You will be attached to the past, fearful and superstitious, and prone to create exactly what you fear most.

Soma (above the third eye, at the hairline): Spiritual connection

Attachments: 'Lost souls', walk-ins. When this chakra is stuck open it is all too easy for spirits to attach. It can be used to detach the etheric body and help the soul move out at death.

Past life chakras (behind the ears along the bony ridge of the skull): Past experiences

Attachments: Past life personas, soul fragments, thought forms from previous beliefs. If the chakras are stuck open, you will feel unsafe and overwhelmed by past life memories of trauma, violent death and fears which leave the way open for past life personas and thought forms to attach or remanifest.

Crown: Spiritual connection

Attachments: Spiritual entities, lost souls, mentors. If it is stuck open, then you will be prey to illusions and false communicators as it leaves you vulnerable to thought forms, spirit attachment or undue influence.

Soul star (above your head): Spiritual enlightenment/ illumination

Attachments: Ancestral spirits, ETs, 'lost souls'. Stuck open or blocked closed, disturbances here may lead to soul fragmentation, spirit attachment, ET invasion, or overwhelm by ancestral spirits.

Stellar gateway (above the soul star): Cosmic doorway to other worlds

Attachments: So-called enlightened beings that are anything but. When it is stuck open, it may be a source of cosmic disinformation which leads to illusion, delusion, deception and disintegration that leaves you totally unable to function in the everyday world.

Causal vortex (above and behind the head): The record of the soul's journey

Attachments: Past life and cultural or ancestral beliefs and soul imperatives.

Alta major (inside the head): Expanding awareness

Attachments: Memories from the past, ancestral and karmic imperatives.
Quick fix: Sweep with Anandalite from the ground up and over the front of your body, over your head, and down to the floor at the back, and back again. Then from side to side and back again.

To Check the Chakras for Attachments

Crystals can be used to 'clean out' hooks or attachments from the chakras. Flint, raw Charoite, Brandenberg, Lemurian Seed, Clear Quartz Points and Stibnite work well if you do not have Anandalite. Simply spiral the crystal in to check the position of the attachment or hook (counterclockwise is usual but use which works for you). Then spiral the crystal out to pull out the attachments or release the hooks. Cleanse the crystal thoroughly and then spiral in light to seal where the attachment was held:

To unwind an attachment or clear a hook

- Beginning with the stellar gateway about a foot and a half above the top of the head (or as high as your arm can reach) and using a clear Quartz, Brandenberg, Anandalite™, Flint, raw Charoite, Smoky Quartz or Selenite crystal – or a Stibnite wand if the attachment is extraterrestrial – 'unwind' the chakra (this is usually done in an anticlockwise direction but do it in the way that feels right to you as not all chakras rotate in the same direction). Wind out in a spiral at least a foot and probably more away from the body.

- When you are sure the chakra is clear and has no attachments, cleanse the crystal by spraying with Petaltone Clear2Light and/or Z14 and then wind it back in the opposite direction.

- Work down each chakra in turn not forgetting the earth star chakra beneath your feet.

- Then wrap yourself – and the person you are working on if you are facilitating the cleanse for someone else – in a cloak of light or Anandalite.

- Then check out the auric field with your mind or the crystal to ensure there is no attachment or influence elsewhere. If there is, disperse it with the crystal and call in light to heal and seal it.

See also spleen chakra page 149 and cord cutting, page 182.

Opening and Integrating the Chakras

A simple crystal layout will cleanse and open the personal chakras so that the lesser known can then be integrated into the system and the whole system run as one.

Personal Chakra Cleanse, Balance and Recharge

- Place Smoky Quartz or other earth star crystal between and slightly below your feet. Picture light and energy radiating out from the crystal into the earth star for two or three minutes and be aware that the chakra is being cleansed and its spin regulated.
- Place Red Jasper or other base chakra crystal on the base chakra. Picture light and energy radiating out from the crystal into the base chakra as before.
- Place Orange Carnelian or other sacral chakra crystal on your sacral chakra, just below the navel, see the light and feel the cleansing process.
- Place Yellow Jasper or other solar plexus crystal on your solar plexus.

- Place Green Aventurine or other heart chakra crystal on your heart.
- Place Blue Lace Agate or other throat chakra crystal on your throat.
- Place Sodalite or other third eye chakra crystal on your brow.
- Place Amethyst or other crown chakra crystal on your crown.
- Breathe deeply taking the breath all the way down to your feet as you inhale, and then letting your attention come slowly up your body as you exhale until you reach your crown. Repeat several times.
- Remain still and relaxed, breathing deep down into your belly and counting to seven before you exhale. As you breathe in and hold, feel the energy of the crystals re-energizing the chakras and from there radiating out through your whole being.
- Now take your attention slowly from the soles of your feet up the midline of your body, feeling how each chakra has become balanced and harmonized.
- When you feel ready, gather your crystals up, starting from the crown. As you reach the earth chakra, be aware of a grounding cord anchoring you to the Earth and into your physical body.
- Cleanse your stones thoroughly (see page 21).

Integrating the lesser-known chakras

Once the personal chakras are up and running efficiently, introduce the lesser-known chakras such as the Gaia gateway, knees and the dantien into the above layout, placing an appropriate crystal. When the lesser-known chakras have been cleansed and activated, allow the energy to flow and be incorporated into the personal chakra alignment and out into the auric field.

[Extracted from *Crystal Prescriptions volume 4*]

The Spleen Protector

If you feel exhausted in someone's company, or wilt when they phone, and especially if you have an ache under your left armpit, then they are drawing on your energy field via the spleen chakra. A spleen protector soon sorts out energy pirates and as a general rule, green crystals such as Jade, Fluorite and Gaspeite work well for the spleen chakra.
Judy Hall, *Complete Crystal Workshop*

The spleen chakra is an area of vulnerability that is often overlooked. This is where the energy vampires or past partners hook into your energy field.

The Spleen Chakra: self-protection and empowerment

Location: A hand's breadth below the left armpit extending down towards the waist, back and front.

When this chakra is wide open, other people can draw on your energy, leaving you depleted particularly at the immune and vitality levels. If you have a constant ache under your left armpit then the chakra is too open and a psychic vampire has hooked in to get their energy fix. Or a past partner is still drawing on the connection no matter how long ago it occurred. When the chakra is blocked, emotional energy especially anger can become stuck there and this will also deplete you.

Overactive/blown/spin too fast: If this chakra is wide open then anyone can hook into your energy and deplete you. You will pick up other people's feelings, especially anger and irritation which may lead to physical pain. You will remain connected to anyone with whom you have had close contact. People can easily take advantage of you, manipulating and coercing you into self-destructive actions that are not for your highest good. Your body may well turn in to attack itself leading to autoimmune diseases. Uncontrollable anger is common when this chakra is blown as you unconsciously rebel against being subtly manipulated or vampirised.

Underactive/blocked/spin too slow: When this chakra is blocked you will feel rootless, purposeless, exhausted and manipulated, powerless. You may well have anger issues but find it difficult to express your anger. You may also suffer constant irritation, some of which goes back to unresolved past life issues. As with the blown chakra, your body may turn in to attack itself. Intimacy with others is impossible when this chakra is locked shut.

Signs that the spleen chakra has hooks in it: Pain under the arm and along the ribs on the left-hand side of the body, a tugging sensation under the arm, lack of energy, absolute exhaustion, someone else becomes more bouncy and alive in your presence.

There is a corresponding chakra on the right side of the body, over the liver. If, having removed hooks from your spleen chakra, you get a pain under the right armpit this is the result of an energy vampire becoming frustrated at having the power source cut off. This can be easily be dealt with (see next page). This closing of the energy portal cuts off energy vampires among the living as well as those who have passed over but not let go.

Closing and protecting the spleen energy portal

Keeping your spleen chakra free from hooks should be a regular part of your spiritual and energetic house-keeping. This is quickly achieved with a crystal.

- Cleanse your spleen chakra by spiralling out a Quartz point, Green Aventurine, Flint, raw Charoite or Rainbow Mayanite to clear any hooks or energetic connections from the chakra, or use a Jasper or Sard tie-cutter.
- To protect the chakra after cord cutting, tape a Tantalite, Green Aventurine, Green Fluorite or Jade crystal over the spleen chakra, or wear one on a long chain so that it reaches to the end of your breastbone level with the chakra.
- Picture a three-dimensional green pyramid extending down from your armpit to your waist, front and back to protect the spleen.
- If the area under your right armpit then begins to ache, tape a piece of Gaspeite, Tugtupite or Bloodstone over the site and leave in place for

several days until the message is received that you will not be giving away any more of your energy. You can also picture a red three-dimensional pyramid protecting this area.

The Auric Field

If your auric field, the biomagnetic energy body that surrounds your physical body, is in any way torn or wounded or carries memories and vulnerabilities via the bio-memory or engrams (see below) or the collective unconscious, you will be vulnerable to invasion or psychic attack.

To understand how subtle bodies work, it helps if we imagine ourselves as a wave on the ocean. Our physical body is the very peak of that wave. Going deeper into the wave itself, we move away from the experience of time and space and the physical limitations of the body and into a broader definition of who we are, our emotions and our thoughts. If we go deeper still, a point is eventually reached where the edges of one wave cannot be differentiated from others: it stops being an individual wave and becomes part of the ocean.

Simon and Sue Lilly, *Crystal Healing*

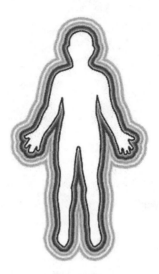

The auric bodies. Coloured fields of light that interplay and interweave.

The physical body is surrounded and interpenetrated by subtle energy fields or 'bodies' that are usually called the aura or biomagnetic sheath. These bodies are linked through, but not limited to, specific chakras. The bodies are like blueprints that hold information, bio-memories and engrams from which the physical body will be constructed. The blueprints affect how the chakras function as well as physical, emotional and mental well-being. In some cases, blockages in the chakras will need to be released by healing the subtle energy body first. In other cases, clearing the chakra will result in a clearing of the subtle energy body. Medical science is slowly recognizing the existence of these bio-memory blueprints.

Bio-memories are memories that are locked into our cells. They carry hereditary memories, past-life memories and memories that have become part of the very fiber of our current personality through constant repetition for years. Both physical and mental patterns can become part of our bio-memory. Bio-memories have the power to trigger physical actions like fight or flight. Mental states like depression and anxiety can quickly become part of our bio-memory if we are not careful. Bio-memories are not only unconscious, but are usually untraceable to any particular source incident.

Original copyright holder unascertainable

These bio-memories are also known as engrams, or engraved memories, and are:

biochemical changes that occur in neural tissues as the result of a powerful or persistent reaction to any situation. An engram is not an ordinary memory, but more like a photograph of the situation or event, complete with the emotional response that accompanied it. Engrams exist just below the level of our consciousness, influencing our emotional responses without our knowledge.

However, engrams are not just found in the physical body and in the 'junk DNA' (see *Crystal Prescriptions volume 6*). They also exist in the subtle bodies. You can picture these subtle energy bodies with their imprints as radiating out from the body in layers, with the chakras connecting them, each having a finer and more subtle vibration. But they are actually interlinked through multidimensional frequencies and interpenetrate each other. Crystals interact with the chakras and the blueprints to bring the bodies back into an appropriate harmony and equilibrium, and to heal energetic 'holes', energy loss, distortion or imprinted patterns that no longer serve you. Having these subtle bodies balanced and in harmony facilitates the flow of kundalini at higher vibrational levels.

The Energy Bodies

Rather than being seen as separate 'layers' it is better to picture the auric field as interpenetrating bands of light that weave together and carry information into the chakras and out again.

Physical-etheric auric body

The physical subtle body, or etheric blueprint, tends to be close to the physical body and can often be seen with a psychic eye as a white aura around that body. It is a biomagnetic program and holds imprints of past life disease, injuries and beliefs which present life symptoms then reflect. It also holds subtle DNA that can be activated or switched off by behaviour and beliefs, and which in turn affects DNA in the physical body. It is connected through the seven traditional, lower frequency chakras on the body and the soma, past life, alta major and causal vortex.

Emotional auric body

The emotional body is created by emotions and feelings, attitudes, heartbreaks, traumas and dramas, not only in the present life but in previous lives. Emotional dis-ease shows up as dark or distorted patches within the subtle emotional body and the solar plexus and heart chakras. The emotional body may contain engrams, bundles of energy that hold a deeply traumatic or joyful memory picture. Dis-ease in this body may also be reflected in the sacral and base chakras, and the knees and feet which will act out insecurities and fears.

Mental auric body

The mental body is created by thoughts, memories, credos and ingrained beliefs from both the present and previous lives. It is connected particularly strongly through the throat and head chakras but may be reflected in the lower body chakras also. This body holds the imprint of all that has been said or taught by authority figures in the past along with inculcated ideologies and points of view. It may need to be cleared and repro-grammed with perspectives more suitable to the current stage of spiritual growth so that it opens the way for evolution on all levels.

Karmic auric body

The karmic body or blueprint holds the imprint of all previous lives, and the soul plan and purpose for the present life. This means that it contains mental programs, physical imprints, and emotional impressions and beliefs that you hold about yourself, many of which may be contradictory as they will arise from very different experiences in various lives. It may also carry past-their-sell-by-date soul imperatives and contracts together with life plans that require reframing and healing (see *Crystal Prescriptions volume 6*). When the karmic body is healed, evolutionary intent can be actualised. This body is accessed through the past life, alta major and causal vortex chakras but may also affect the soma, knee and earth star.

Ancestral auric body

The ancestral body holds all that you have inherited down your ancestral lines on both sides, everything your ancestors passed on to you either at the physical or more subtle levels through the matrilineal and 'junk DNA'. This may include family sagas, belief systems and attitudes, culture and expectations, traumas and dramas that shape your world. Healing sent back down the ancestral line to the core experience rebounds forward to heal the line going out into the future, making change possible. This body can be accessed through the soul star, past life, alta major, higher heart, earth star and Gaia gateway chakras and may have a great deal to do with how much at home you feel on the planet and whether you are able to put your soul purpose into practice. You may need to release ancestral expectations before soul evolution may occur (see *Crystal Prescriptions volume 6*).

Planetary auric body

While you are in incarnation you also have a subtle

energy body that links into the planet and the Earth's etheric body and meridians. This planetary body is connected to the wider cosmos, the luminaries, planets and stellar bodies and the outer reaches of the universe. Through this planetary body you are therefore connected into the wider whole and the collective unconscious. The planetary body is reflected in your birthchart and is accessed through the past life, alta major, causal vortex, soma, stellar and Gaia gateway chakras. Cosmic or soul dis-ease can be corrected through the planetary subtle body.

Spiritual or Light auric body

The spiritual or lightbody is an integrated, luminous, vibrating energy field consisting of the physical body and all the subtle energy bodies, plus the spirit or soul, connected through all the chakras but especially through the higher dimensional ones: soma, soul star, stellar gateway, Gaia gateway, alta major and causal vortex. It is an electromagnetic field of varying oscillation with integrated frequencies from the highest to the lowest: being light in all its varied manifestations. The body itself resonates with the universe, the universal mind and with your own soul or spirit. When the lightbody is activated, it may literally re-encode your 'junk DNA' bringing out its highest potential and allowing your soul's purpose to manifest.

To instantly harmonize the subtle energy bodies

- Hold a piece of Anandalite or other subtle body harmonizer in your hand and sweep it at arm's length from your feet up over your head and down to your feet at the back – if you find it difficult to reach ask a friend to assist. If the crystal 'sticks' at any one spot, leave it in place until it begins to move of its own volition once more. Then bring it up and over your head again and back to the floor.

- Sweep it from one side of your body to the other moving from your feet up over your head and down to your feet on the other side. Return to the first side.

- You may have to carry out several sweeps moving your arm closer in each time to integrate and harmonize all the subtle bodies with the higher dimensional energetic levels of the chakras.

You can also integrate the chakras and subtle auric bodies with the longer exercise that follows.

Harmonizing the Chakras and Subtle Bodies with Crystals

Cleansing and rebalancing your chakras and maintaining your subtle bodies on a regular basis ensure well-being and protect you against psychic attack. You can either do a complete chakra cleanse and recharge, as below, or you can cleanse one chakra at a time if you particularly identify with the issue or qualities for that chakra or if there is a blockage. If you do one chakra only, you still need to place a detoxifying crystal on the earth star chakra at your feet. Placing crystals on the earth star grounds or discharges toxic energies, and reminds you to keep your physical body connected to the Earth. This cleanse-and-recharge will be particularly important as your energies shift to a higher vibration and new higher chakras come online.

You can quickly check whether a chakra is open and functioning optimally by using a pendulum (see page 16). Check the energetic state of your subtle bodies in the same way.

A simple but effective layout for bringing your body back into balance is to place a cleansed and activated crystal over each of your chakras – you can dowse or intuit which crystals are suitable, or follow the colours given below. But don't be afraid to use your intuition or dowsing, as 'chakra colours' are not necessarily the traditional rainbow arc. There are other crystals that may be more appropriate. Check which of the minor chakras should be included (see diagram on page 121). Place an appropriate stone on each chakra and leave in place for 20–30 minutes. This layout is best done lying down so that you can place crystals below your feet and above your head.

Basic rebalancing and aligning layout

- Place a Gaia gateway crystal about arm's length below your feet.
- Place Smoky Quartz, Flint, Hematite or other earth star crystal between and slightly below your feet. Picture light and energy radiating out from the crystal into the earth star chakra for two or three minutes and be aware that the chakra is being cleansed, its spin regulated, and its function re-energized.
- Place Red Jasper, Carnelian or other appropriate crystal on the base chakra. Picture light and energy radiating out from the crystal into the base chakra before moving through the physical body in a cleansing and revitalizing wave.
- Place Orange Carnelian, Golden or Orange Calcite or other appropriate crystal on your sacral chakra, just below the navel. Picture the radiating light and

feel the cleansing and energizing process in the chakra and then through the subtle energy bodies.

- Place Yellow Jasper, Citrine or other appropriate crystal on your solar plexus. Picture the radiating light and feel the cleansing and energizing process in the chakra and then through the emotional body.

- Place Green Aventurine, Rose Quartz or other appropriate crystal on your heart. Picture the radiating light and feel the cleansing and energizing process in the chakra and then through the subtle energy bodies.

- Place Blue Lace Agate, Lapis Lazuli or other appropriate crystal on your throat. Picture the radiating light and feel the cleansing and energizing process in the chakra and then through the mental body.

- Place Sodalite, Apophyllite or other appropriate crystal on your brow. Picture the radiating light and feel the cleansing and energizing process in the chakra and then in the subtle energy bodies.

- Place Amethyst, Quartz or other appropriate crystal on your crown. Picture the radiating light and feel the cleansing and energizing process in the chakra and then in your spiritual body.

- Place an Anandalite or other appropriate crystals on the soul star and stellar gateway chakras above your head.

- Now take your attention slowly from the soles of your feet up the midline of your body feeling how each chakra has become balanced and harmonized, and how each is connected to an energy body into which the crystal radiates its energy.

- Feel how the Gaia gateway and the stellar gateway chakras also connect around the edges of your aura in addition to the line up the spine. Your auric field is connected by protective, integrative crystal energy.

- Remain still and relaxed, breathing deep down into your belly and counting to seven before you exhale.

- Once again, take your mind down to the chakras beneath your feet and work up through each chakra again in turn. As you breathe in and hold, feel the energy of the re-energized chakra radiating out through your subtle bodies bringing each one into deeper alignment with the others and with your physical body. You will build layer on layer of replenished and rebalanced subtle bodies so that your whole aura is in balance. If at any time you feel a blockage, simply breathe the light of the crystal into the site until it dissolves.

- When you feel ready, gather your crystals up, starting from above your head. As you reach the earth star and Gaia gateway chakras, be aware of the grounding cord anchoring you to the Earth and into your physical body.

- Cleanse your stones thoroughly (see page 21).

[Extracted and enlarged from *Crystal Prescriptions volume 4*]

Soul Splits, Soul Fragmentation and Soul Loss

Soul loss, sometimes known as a soul split, is a condition that leaves you particularly vulnerable to psychic attack. We are used to thinking of the soul as 'all of a piece' but, as shamans have known for thousands of years, this is not always the case. Souls can energetically split, combine and recombine with other members of an overall soul group, for instance. But souls can also split into two or more 'pieces' and *appear* to be totally different entities (see *Crystal Prescriptions volume 6* for a deeper explanation). It is not uncommon to find that a soul has parts in different physical incarnations at the same time. These parts can be energetically linked even when the vehicles for those soul parts are hundreds of miles apart, or even living in apparently different time frames. It is also quite usual during past life regression to discover that a portion of an overall soul has been left at a traumatic death or other soul-shattering event. Soul loss almost invariably accompanies post traumatic stress disorder (PTSD, see *Crystal Prescriptions volume 6*). Even joyful occasions may still have a fragment of soul attached 'back in time'. Thinking of the soul as a hologram helps in understanding this process. A hologram can be both here and there, split and yet still cohesive. Each tiny fragment reflecting a full picture of the whole. Soul retrieval, bringing together and reintegrating lost soul parts, helps you to feel centred, balanced and whole once more. I pursue this topic in more depth in *Crystal Prescriptions volume 6* but in the meantime here's a brief introduction and an emergency soul retrieval procedure should you need one.

Soul loss

Parts of the overall self may remain at past life deaths, traumatic or joyful moments and so on rather than incarnate with the main soul at birth into the present life. Soul loss may also occur during the current life.

Soul splits, past life and ancestral invasion

Soul loss can also occur when a past life or ancestral persona breaks through and is acted out. Especially if the soul part left in the previous incarnation is still very active. In extreme cases this can feel as though two people are inhabiting the same skin or that you have been taken over by someone else. In *The Book of Why* I quoted the case of Donovan, a Vietnam vet. He was a soul who had a 'foot in both camps'. Although Donovan was apparently living in a present life as an alienated outsider (itself a symptom of soul loss and past life persona breakthrough), he was still also concurrently living an 'old' life in the Vietnam War, which had broken through in spontaneous regression. His soul was split between the two and there was a huge crossover so that Donovan didn't really know where he belonged. He couldn't function properly in his 'present' life because so much of him was 'back there' stuck in a life that was cut short – and so much of 'back there' was operating in his current life. His vivid dreams, recollections and intuitions tried to take him to a point where his soul could reintegrate and heal the past. Had he had a therapist facilitating this, it could have been quicker – and smoother – but 'doing it himself' was a part of the alienated outsider persona he'd carried over and he needed to reach the insights himself. It was a part of his soul intention.

Crystal soul retrieval

Gathering up pieces of the soul so that it can reintegrate has been practised by soul retrieval practitioners throughout aeons of time and it may be extremely helpful in cases where someone does not feel fully present, or in certain psychiatric illnesses. Pieces of a soul may be left earlier in the present life, or in other lives and it is part of soul retrieval or past life therapy to retrieve and reintegrate these fragments as appropriate. Bringing them back through a crystal purifies, heals and re-energizes the soul fragment. However, there are times when reintegrating a soul part is not appropriate, in which case a crystal can act as a container for that soul until it becomes apparent where to direct the soul or putting it into the care of the higher self.

There are many people walking around in a fogged, fragmented and disconnected state as a past life persona has taken over part or all of their present life personality. Soul fragmentation leaves such people open to psychic attack or attachment from 'lost', 'stuck' or 'alien' souls and such like, as well as the breakthrough of another past life persona. Complex soul release, reintegration or past life healing may be required in addition to soul retrieval. This really is a job for an expert (see Resources and page 210 for how to move a stuck soul on in an emergency).

Widely differing past life experiences may create a subtle soul split within an incarnated soul who is apparently all of a piece but is actually experiencing an inner split within the same lifetime. The sexuality-spirituality axis split is common and powerfully affects the ability to be intimate in the present life or to form a parental or other bond. If someone has taken a vow of celibacy in a previous life, for instance, and not rescinded it, it may be re-enacted through a subconscious past life memory borne deep in the soul. The person will feel guilty during a sexual act. But equally, another part of the soul, which has enjoyed sexual engagements in the past, may be pushed to the fore as a reaction against the celibacy. The two personas will battle it out, one appearing uppermost and then the other. Similarly, an ancestor can intrude in something that is stronger than a light spirit attachment. This is particularly so when the ancestor has a vested interest, or unfinished agenda, in certain situations coming to fruition. But in such cases, the 'ancestor' will most probably be an earlier incarnation of the same soul.

Sometimes, however, a soul 'splits' and comes into incarnation in two distinctly separate bodies. This is generally because 'one half' incarnates to assist or facilitate the 'other half' in a specific task. However, soul splits can occur for more traumatic, less deliberately planned, reasons. Some 'soul splits' reintegrate after death, but others continue as separate souls and cannot be reintegrated during the present lifetime. These types of soul split may need the assistance of expert help, but the symptoms and first aid treatment are the same. (*Crystal Prescriptions volume 6* addresses this in more depth.)

Trigonic: the soul midwife crystal

Trigonic crystals, with cascading descending triangles on their faces, are the soul crystal *par excellence*. They hold the record of the soul in all its incarnations wherever and whenever that may have been. A Trigonic keeps track of soul parts located elsewhere and assists them to communicate as a whole. As Trigonics are rare, it is possible to use the Trigonic card from the *Crystal Wisdom Healing Oracle Kit* to effect soul healing.

Signs of soul loss, soul split, or past life or ancestral persona breakthrough

The immediate symptoms of soul loss or the breakthrough of a past life or ancestral persona – which has a similar effect – can be interchangeable with spirit attachment signals (see page 213), but there are additional subtle signals that may take some time to be recognized:

- Feeling vague, nebulous and insubstantial. Somehow 'not there'. To an outside eye, incomplete and fragmented.
- Multiple selves try to make themselves known, with sudden switches and memory loss.
- Problems with time.
- 'Blank' eyes stare into the distance.

- No eye contact.
- 'Someone else' looks out from the eyes.
- A profound sense of disconnection from everyday life.
- Behaviour is out of character with normal persona.
- Obsessive, escapist or addictive behaviour and constant 'busyness' prevail.
- Severe insomnia.
- Constant fears and anxieties.
- Unusual thought patterns, sometimes self-destructive.
- Intense dreams or fantasies with a nightmarish quality.
- Hearing voices.
- A feeling of being controlled by someone else.
- Sudden overwhelming bouts of tiredness or yawning and chronic fatigue.
- Overwhelming sugar cravings.
- Memories of portions of life especially shock or trauma have been blocked out.
- Prolonged periods of depression.
- PTSD (post traumatic stress disorder).
- Trust is missing. Everyone is kept at arm's length, no vulnerability even to close friends or family.
- A profound numbness invades every part of life. Issues are not recognized or dealt with.
- Feeling like a different person after a shock or traumatic life event.
- Psychosomatic dis-eases are present.

- Severe disappointment in life.
- A deep sense of unworthiness prevails.
- A 'dark night of the soul' is constantly undergone.
- There is no sense of purpose or meaning in life.
- Things are done because they have to be done. There is no joy or purpose in it.
- Overexcitement, constantly 'revved up'.
- Being on an emotional or mental 'high'.
- Rapid, constant and somewhat random chatter.
- Longing for a sense of being an authentic self.

Soul loss, cravings and addictions

Soul loss, soul splits and spirit attachment may all have addiction or cravings as a characteristic 'symptom' or indication of the condition. Something is felt to be missing, at the emotional or spiritual level. The soul tries to 'fill the gap' with a substitute or, in cases of spirit attachment, the attaching spirit seeks to get the hit to which it was addicted in its former life. Crystals can assist in filling the gap. See A–Z Directory page 335 and *Crystal Prescriptions volume 6* for further solutions.

Healing a Soul Split and Returning a Soul Fragment

This layout calls home and integrates soul fragments that are ready to return and heal or soul splits. Healing a soul split in this way is only applicable when both parts of the soul are contained within a single human being – even though they may be behaving as though they are separate individuals. It is not suitable for cases where there are two different physical bodies involved (that has to wait until at least one has passed beyond death of the physical body). Calling on your higher self to assist facilitates the process. Dowse to ascertain which would be the best crystals for you. Have a Selenite crystal to hand in case you need a container for a soul fragment that is not yet ready to reintegrate. In this exercise there is nothing to do, simply allow the process to take place.

Higher self

The 'higher self' is the part of ourself that is not fully in incarnation and, therefore, has a much clearer picture of why we are here and where we are going. It carries the memory of our previous lives, our soulplan – and our soul overlays and soul splits. It constantly monitors the whole of the soul, whether fragmented or not. The higher self acts as guide, mentor and information assistant to the soul in incarnation. It is a useful guide to facilitate soul retrieval.

Soul retrieval exercise

- Cleanse and balance your chakras as far as possible.
- Ensure that you are in a quiet, protected space.
- Place a Trigonic Quartz, Shiva Shell, Preseli Bluestone or other soul retrieval crystal on your soma chakra (mid-hairline just above the third eye).
- Place an Anandalite, Trigonic or other soul retrieval crystal on your heart seed chakra (base of your breastbone below the heart chakra).
- With the fingers of each hand, tap either side of your breastbone with the first finger about a hand's breath below your collarbone on the 'spirit ground' points on the illustration below. If it feels appropriate you can also tap these points, the 'sore spots' and the 'baggage points' with a small Trigonic, Brandenberg or Lemurian Seed crystal.

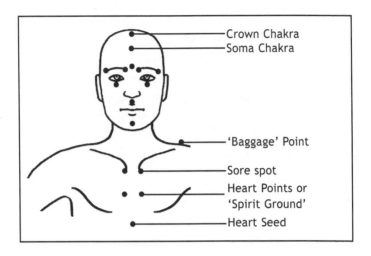

Crown Chakra
Soma Chakra
'Baggage' Point
Sore spot
Heart Points or 'Spirit Ground'
Heart Seed

- Ask your higher self to call back to you any soul fragments that are ready to return, or to repair a split soul if this is appropriate. Request your higher self to ensure that only fragments that rightfully belong with your soul *at the present moment* will return to you.

- The soul fragments will pass through the crystals to purify and re-energize them as they reintegrate, leaving the past behind them but bringing forward any wisdom learned. As the soul part returns, absorb it along with the crystal energy into every cell of your body and at all energetic levels. Feel the light carried in the crystal healing and reintegrating your whole being.

- As the soul part returns, absorb it along with the crystal energy into every cell of your body and at all energetic levels. Feel the light carried in the crystal healing and reintegrating your whole being.

- If a soul portion is not yet ready to reintegrate, place it in the Selenite crystal. When the exercise is complete, ask if it is more appropriate to send that soul part to the care of the higher self for the time being. If so, ask the crystal to release the soul part into the care of your higher self. If it prefers to remain in the crystal for the time being, check out every few days what the appropriate action is for that soul part. It may be that it stays with the higher self for the duration of the current life.
- When the integration is complete, pass Anandalite or Selenite round your whole aura to heal and seal it once again.

Disconnecting

Many people walk around with a dark cloud of energy that is not 'theirs' all around them. This may lead to energy depletion, illness or your life falling apart. Keeping your energy safe and contained means only opening connections with other people when it is appropriate to do so – and closing them afterwards. This is especially true if you work with clients. If you have regular appointments or work metaphysically with people, it is vital that you set up a 'disconnection signal' at the end of each slot so that you do not carry any energy, dis-ease or emotion that is not yours away with you, and to ensure that your client leaves nothing behind them. A disconnection signal can be as simple as shaking hands or closing the door. If you move from person to person, consciously leave each one behind as you close the door or step away. Let that be the signal to your unconscious mind that you are now letting that person go. However, a large Smoky Quartz crystal near to the door which you touch after they have left can be extremely useful as can 'combing' your aura with Flint or a raw Charoite shard.

Exercise: Disconnecting

- Take two or three good deep breaths, pick up a large Green Aventurine or Smoky Quartz crystal and then place it down again firmly. Check that your spleen is disconnected (see page 149 and if necessary protect it with a green pyramid and remove any cords).

If the person was particularly troubled or stressed, you may also want to spray the room, or yourself, with Clear2Light Essence, or Earthlight or other clearing spray.

Vows, Promises, Pacts and Soul Contracts

Many people are unwittingly manipulated by promises made in the past (whenever that past may have been). These promises may have been to another person: "I'll always love you", "always be there for you", "never let you go" and so on; or to yourself: "I'll get even", "I'll never forget" or "I'll never let him/her go", all of which are equally debilitating. Or they may have been carried by the ancestral line (see *Crystal Prescriptions volume 6*). 'Forever' is an exceedingly long time, encompassing incarnations in many different dimensions. You may have made a soul contract in the between-life state that holds you fast but which is no longer possible or appropriate. Promises in other lives bind the souls together throughout many lifetimes and may be inappropriate in the present life. But vows work equally potently when they have been made earlier in the present life; you do not need to believe in reincarnation to be affected by previous promises. People may also be held by vows such as to celibacy or poverty, which may create difficulties in a present life relationship. Vows that were made to you may also be inappropriate and may need to be dissolved or renegotiated as otherwise they could lead to vulnerabilities and manipulation.

Exercise: Renegotiating a vow

- Place yourself in a crystal bubble and hold an appropriate crystal (see A–Z Directory).
- When you are relaxed and ready, picture the person in your mind and say firmly and clearly, out loud, "I hereby rescind all vows, promises, pacts, arrangements and soul contracts that I have made in this or any other life, or in the between-life state, that are no longer appropriate and no longer serve me. I set myself free. I also set free anyone from whom I have exhorted a vow or promise anywhere in the past."
- Put the crystal down firmly and clap your hands together loudly to signify the end of those vows.
- Cleanse the crystal thoroughly.
- Stamp your feet firmly on the ground, and walk forward freed from the old vows and promises.
- A Green Aventurine taped under your left armpit for a week or two, or a Gaspeite or Tugtupite on the right side, may be required until the message has been accepted.

If you are non-visual: Hold a cleansed and dedicated piece of Pietersite or Leopardskin Jasper and state that you are now released from all former vows, promises and pacts that you have made in this or any other life.

For a more specific method: See *Crystal Prescriptions volume 6* or *Good Vibrations*.

Crystal Cord Cutting

We have already seen how cords and hooks from other people can link into your chakras, sometimes still remaining long after a relationship of one kind or another has passed its sell-by date. Death and transition to another state of being may have little effect on the hooks and subtle energy imprints that have been left behind. Karmic enmeshment may also tie you to another person, but the source is way back in the past. Fortunately release may be effected in the present. Cutting the cords facilitates letting go of all the oughts, shoulds and if-onlys which make our contact with other people conditional and which hold us, and them, back from developing as people in our own right. This cord cutting has positive, beneficial results for both parties.

Cord cutting is extremely effective, especially when supplemented with crystals. The following exercise uses the power of visualization, seeing things in your mind's eye. But some people will never 'see' anything because they use a different mode of perception such as kinaesthetic 'sensing' or 'feeling'. If you find it difficult to visualize you could find a place outside in nature where you can physically draw the two circles: in sand, on grass or even on concrete. Use a line in the dirt, chalk, spray paint, rice, small pebbles, anything that will delineate your space (and see *if you are non-visual* below). Then sweep the crystal all around yourself. It is more important that you *feel* the subtle energies and cords releasing than it is to visualize them. The crystals will assist you in this. Allow them to point out to you where the hooks and cords are. These may well be some distance out from your physical body so sweep well out and way above your head. The crystal will linger at any place that needs additional attention. Remember to heal and seal each place with an appropriate crystal – or crystal light in the interim.

Exercise: Cord cutting visualization

- Choose your crystal from the cord cutting entry in the A–Z Directory (page 277). Shards of Flint or raw Charoite are ideal. Have an aura-sealing crystal ready as well (see page 262).

- Take time to relax and settle, breathing gently. Slowly raise and lower your eyelids ten times and then leave them closed. Without opening your eyes, raise them to the point between and slightly above your eyebrows as this helps images to form.

- Then picture yourself walking in a meadow or other favourite place such as a beach on a nice, warm, sunny day. Really let yourself feel the grass or the sand beneath your feet, the cool earth or the water below. There is a gentle breeze playing around your face, keeping you cool and comfortable.

- Spend a little time exploring your meadow and then choose the spot where you want to do this work.

- Draw a circle around yourself as you stand in the meadow. The circle should be at arm's length and go right around you. You could use paint, chalk, light or whatever comes to mind. This circle delineates your space. (If you use a hoop of light, it can be pulled up around you if needed.)

- In front of you, close to but not touching your circle, draw another circle the same size. Picture the person with whom you wish to cut the ties in the circle. (If you have difficulty in seeing the person clearly, you could picture a photograph being placed in the circle.) Do not let the circles overlap; peg them down if necessary.

- Explain to the person why you are doing this exercise. Tell them that you are not cutting off any unconditional love there may be, but that you wish to be free from the old emotional conditioning, karma and bonds that built up in the past, and any expectations in the present.

- Look to see how the ties symbolically manifest themselves. Then, using your cord cutting crystal, spend time removing them, first from yourself healing and sealing the places where they were with crystal light, then removing them from the other person. Make sure you get all the cords, especially the ones around the back that you may overlook and those that are far out in your subtle etheric bodies. Sweep the crystal well out from your aura and then slowly work in towards your physical body. Pile the ties up outside the circle.

- Check out the higher chakras above your head. If you have problems with cords at high vibrational levels, ask your higher self and the crystal to deal with these on your behalf. Hold the crystal above your head and mentally hand it over and allow the process to complete.

- When you are sure you have cleared all the cords, and sealed all the places where they have been, let unconditional love, forgiveness and acceptance (where possible) flow between you and the other person. Then let that other person go back to where they belong. Into their own space. (If you experience problems with this, use the portal crystals on page 223 to seal the portal behind them.)

- Mentally gather up all the cords and find an appropriate way of destroying them. You may wish to visualize a large bonfire on to which you throw them, or a swiftly flowing river into which you cast them. Make sure you have destroyed all the cords.

- If you are using a fire, move nearer to the flames and feel the transmuted energy warming, purifying, healing and energizing you and your crystal, filling all the empty spaces left by removing the cords. This is your own creative life force coming back to you in its transmuted and purified form. Absorb as much of this energy as you can. If you feel able to, move into the fire and become like the phoenix, reborn from the flames.

- If you have water in your visualization, you might like to enter the water, or to use the heat of the sun to purify, heal and energize yourself and your crystal. Then wrap a bubble of crystal light around you to protect yourself.

- Then sweep an aura-sealing crystal such as Anandalite all around yourself. Use it to pull your aura into a sensible distance all around you.

- When you have completed all the cutting you wish to do, open your eyes and bring your attention back into the room. Allow yourself plenty of time to readjust, breathing more deeply and bringing yourself into full awareness with feet firmly on the ground. Have a hot drink to bring you fully back into your body and the present moment.

If you are non-visual: Place two photographs (or write the name of the person with whom you wish to cut the cords) within two circles that do not touch – you can use a large dinner plate for this. Place coloured thread or a net (the kind that fruit is wrapped in is ideal) or whatever your imagination tells you would be appropriate to link them. Using your crystal, carefully remove the threads from your picture and then from the other person. Burn them to transmute the energy. Place a piece of Anandalite, Rose Quartz or other aura-sealing crystal on each photograph and allow its healing energy to seal the places where the cords were located. Then move the circles wide apart, certainly into another room and preferably out of your space entirely. If you were using a piece of paper with a name written on it, this can be burnt with loving compassion and forgiveness.

In an emergency

Sweep all around your body with a shard of Flint, raw Charoite, Anandalite or other cord cutting crystal, asking that all ties will be removed and the site healed. Allow the hooks and cords to go back to the source. Then ask that any hooks or cords you yourself have placed into the other person's energy field be retracted and the place sealed.

Taking Back the Heart

People unthinkingly give their heart to others. But few realise how devastating the effects of leaving their heart in someone else's keeping can be – or the effects of having it 'stolen' by a needy or manipulative person. Nor how long the process may last as it can span lives. Not having a fully functioning, open heart can literally be soul shattering. Handing your heart over to another, having your heart shackled to a memory, suffering from a 'broken heart' or being 'hard-hearted' is almost certainly linked to past and present heartache and will certainly create psychic vulnerability and most probably physical dis-ease if not healed.

Signs that the heart has been lost, stolen or broken

No passion to life	Defensive	Guilty	Naive
No fire and zest	Sacrificial	Scared	Cynical
Takes but does not give	Remote	Bitter	Fearful
Life has lost its colour	Burned-out	Alienated	Greedy
Defines self by roles	Dissociated	Separate	Judgmental
Unavailable for relationship	Selfish	Needy	Cruel

Afraid of intimacy	Jealous	Possessive	Control-freak
Commitment-phobic	Promiscuous	Dishonest	Unavailable
Cold patch over heart	Manipulative	Deceitful	Insincere

(*after Chuck Spezzano, augmented by Judy Hall, extracted from* The Soulmate Myth)

Most of these states are, of course, emotional in origin. Defensiveness, for instance, arises when you have been hurt and feel the need to protect your heart, but so too does cynicism. Burnout occurs when you have given unceasingly, but have not allowed yourself to be nurtured in return, or have been unable to find unconditional love. A broken heart may well lie behind a tendency to define yourself by the role of 'parent', 'wife', 'husband' or 'loner'. The net result of a wounded heart is that life loses its zest and passion, and your auric bodies become transparent and 'ragged' and your heart chakra out of balance. A desperate soul whose heart is pained may well be both needy and greedy, but could well become judgmental or bitter, seeking revenge. Fortunately it is easy to reclaim your heart. Danburite is an excellent crystal to support claiming back your heart.

Visualization: Reclaiming your heart

- Holding a healing heartache crystal, relax and focus your attention on your heart. Feel its beat; hear its sounds. As you listen to the rhythm of your heart and feel its pulsating energy, allow yourself to relax a little deeper. Slowly, let your heart transport you into another time and space.

- You find yourself standing in the temple of your inner heart. Its colour and dimensions are unique to you. Explore this temple. Notice if its walls are ruined or broken. Notice if you meet anyone else (if so, remember to work with them in a moment). Recognize if there are heartstrings pulling you in a certain direction. If there are, use a cord cutting crystal to cut the connection and then heal and seal this place with golden crystal light.

- You may already have become aware of someone who holds your heart; if so picture that person standing before you. If you have not yet recognized who holds your heart, ask to be shown this right now. (If there is more than one person, work on one at a time.)

- You see that this person holds a portion of your heart. It may appear symbolically. If so, look at its colour, shape and form. You may find that it is freely offered back to you, or you may find that the person wants to hold on to it. If they do so, ask their reason. They may well feel that they have to look after you, or you may have made them a promise, or you may have given your heart into their keeping. State firmly that it is now time to reclaim your heart. If necessary thank them, release them, release yourself, whatever is appropriate.

- Now take a deep breath and focus all your intention. Firmly and clearly, reach out and take this heart back. Say out loud: "I take back all that is mine and I freely give you back all that is yours." You may need to purify your heart before taking it back if it holds the other person's energy. If so, see it coming back to you through a cloud of pink light or a Rose Quartz or other heart healing crystal.

- Welcome your heart back with love and place it once more within you. (You may like to place a piece of Rose Quartz or Rhodochrosite over your heart to symbolise this return.)

- [If you experience any problems, ask for a guide, a helper, your higher self or an angelic being to come to your assistance.]

- Repeat this reclaiming until there is no one left who holds a part of your heart and your heart is whole once more. Check that you yourself do not inadvertently hold a piece of someone else's heart. If you do, then surrender it willingly and allow it to return to where it belongs. Then check the inner temple of your heart once again. You will probably find that it is looking much better. You may well find that the symbolic pieces of your heart decorate the walls. If it needs any further repair, use crystal light or place a crystal over your heart.

- Take a few moments to open your heart and offer forgiveness to the other person and, if appropriate, allow yourself to receive their forgiveness and place it in your heart. Open yourself to divine love or to crystal energy and fill your heart from that source.

- Now consciously step out of that inner temple, but know that it is within your own heart, which is now whole and healed. Become aware of your breathing once again, and the beat of your heart. Slowly bring your attention back into the room. Take your attention down to your feet and ground yourself firmly with your grounding cord. Picture a bubble of light enclosing you, sealing your energies, so that you are safe and contained. When you are ready, open your eyes. After a few moments of reflection, get up and move around the room.

If you are non-visual: Place Danburite, Smoky Brandenberg Amethyst or other heart chakra crystal over your heart. Say out loud: "I call back any pieces of my heart that I may have given or had stolen away, no matter how inadvertently or lovingly this may have occurred. I claim back my heart now." Leave the crystal in place until your heart feels whole and healed once more.

[Extracted from *Good Vibrations*]

Immune Stimulator Layout

Oriental Medicine calls viruses and bacteria "evil spirits" because they come in from the outside unbidden, they can invade through physical wounds, and they are only able to get in if the immune system is not strong enough to find and eliminate them. Likewise, "dark energies" seem to be able to infect a person when their emotional body has been wounded.

http://souldetective.net/2011/06/detrimental-energies/

A damaged immune system leaves you vulnerable to psychic invasion. Your immune systems – physical and subtle – act as protectors for your bioenergy, endocrine and hormonal systems in addition to your physical body. One of the most effective ways to keep your energy strong is to use the healing and immune stimulator layout below. This layout works at both the physical and the more subtle psychic immune system level to give you physical and metaphysical stimulation and protection. Remember to cleanse and dedicate crystals before use, and cleanse afterwards.

Immune Grid

- Place six Quantum Quattro, Smithsonite or Bloodstones charged with the intention to provide ongoing healing and immune system stimulation around your bed, either under the bed itself or under the mattress.
- Place two at head height, two at the middle of the breastbone and two at the feet.
- Leave them in place remembering to cleanse them regularly.

Alternatively: Lie on the floor and grid the crystals around you for 20 minutes. Then wear an immune stimulator crystal over your higher heart chakra (see A–Z Directory).

Depression Release

Depression is a debilitating condition that can leave you wide open to psychic attack, spirit attachment and soul loss as well as vulnerability to thought forms, transgenerational imperatives and the like. This release is an adaption of an exercise given to me by Nina of *Gemworld* to accompany Magdalena Stone. Magdalena is a tumbled Witches Finger: a potent cleansing brew of Smokey Quartz, Rutile, Tourmaline, Chlorite, Amphibole and Hematite. The tumbling transforms the somewhat jagged energy of a Witches Finger into something much smoother. It is said that Witches Finger gives support and "helps one to see and overcome the darker side of one's nature, one's shadow self". As it is rather rare and the gentler Magdalena Stone is difficult to source, I adapted the exercise to use with antidepression stones such as Amethyst, Kunzite or Lepidolite. Using a grounding and detoxifying crystal at your feet during the exercise enhances it, making the release more powerful. Choose a crystal with which you resonate from the A–Z Directory (see page 280).

The Depression Release

- Place a Flint, Smoky Quartz, Obsidian, Shungite or other detoxifying crystal between or beneath your feet depending on the size of the crystal. A large crystal on which you can rest your feet is ideal but two smaller ones, one under each foot, works well.

- Hold a depression-healing crystal such as Kunzite in your hand. Allow the crystal to take your hand to wherever a release is needed to let go of the source of your depression.

- Close your eyes and look up to above and between your eyebrows to encourage images to form. Picture yourself walking into a warm, turquoise-blue sea.

- As you go deeper, imagine you have your feet firmly embedded on the sea floor.

- All around you is dark and you are enveloped in a density you can't see beyond. As you work with the energy of Magdalena or other crystal, feel the negative depressed energy draining down through your feet and into the detoxifying crystal. You will be released from the cloying anchor that has been trapping you and you will slowly rise through the layers of darkness.

- The release of the depressed energy has now been transformed into something more hopeful and comforting, and you can see beyond the darkness. You rise up through the sea towards the light above. This brings clarity into your life and helps you focus on your goals, which are now achievable, taking away confusion and bringing confidence and the ability to make decisions.

- As you break through the surface, the sunshine is on your face and you are connected to the Universal Energy. If you work with the guidance of Angels, ask them to be with you as you walk forward into the light.

- Check that your boundaries are strong, pull your aura into a sensible distance around you (not more than arm's length, no closer than your elbow).

- Cleanse the crystals thoroughly and keep the Magdalena, Kunzite or other antidepression stone close to you. Hold it over your heart if ever you feel yourself sinking down into depression again.

Alternatively: Place five Auralite 23 or Amethyst points (points facing in) around your head and a Smoky Quartz point down at your feet. Lie in the crystals for 5–15 minutes.

Overcoming Ill Wishing or Psychic Attack

Psychic protection is most often needed when you come under ill wishing or psychic attack or when you have a spirit attachment (see page 212). Ill wishing is a concentrated shaft of ill will or vitriolic, jealous thought that does you harm. It may be triggered inadvertently by malicious, destructive or vindictive thoughts, but it may be consciously and intensely directed, in which case it is called psychic attack. Much of this ill wishing is unwitting simply because people do not recognize the power of thought. Ill wishing also happens when you send out harmful or toxic thoughts to another person.

Ill wishing is common in relationships that break up and one person agonises over the situation, or vows to get even or to get the person back (if you are on the receiving end, put a green or yellow pyramid around your spleen now). Any powerful emotion can create ill wishing, which may come from the living and the 'dead'. Psychic attack is a more serious form of ill wishing in which the sender deliberately invokes harm but psychic attack can be dealt with in the same way as ill wishing.

Protection against ill wishing comes from having positive thoughts focused on how well protected and safe you are. Being mindful and staying in the moment rather than dwelling on negative possibilities helps enormously, as does a sense of humour. If you can laugh at people and their antics they are unlikely to cause you harm. If you are someone who broods over perceived slights, change your thinking!

Subtle attack indications

- Total, sudden energy drain
- Accident prone
- Waking suddenly in the night
- Life not working
- Constant illness
- Debilitating fatigue
- Feeling of invasion
- Feeling of being watched
- Body pain – sudden and sharp or continuous dull ache
- Incessant negative thoughts that are not yours
- Panic attacks
- Nightmares
- Fear of being alone
- Sugar, chocolate or alcohol cravings

Ill wishing works by:

- The power of suggestion

- Fear
- Energetic weakness
- Intention

The most potent effects of ill wishing can arise not from the perpetrator, however, but from your own mind. An overactive imagination, together with the power of thought, is a fearsome weapon and we often wield it against ourselves. Ill wishing is heightened when:

- Someone has made a threat against you of which you are aware.
- You know you have been 'cursed'.
- You believe: "I am vulnerable and have no protection against this."
- You feel that the person concerned is stronger than you are.
- You do not trust yourself.
- You have given away your power.

So, one of the most effective defences against ill wishing is to feel invulnerable, invincible and fearless – but not in an egotistical way. It is more a sense of quiet, inner confidence that you are safe. Wearing Eye of the Storm (Judy's Jasper) over your higher heart chakra increases your sense of inner safety.

Dealing with Psychic Attack from an Unknown Source

If you don't know where an attack is coming from, take suitable precautions:

- Put yourself in a crystal bubble and strengthen your auric field with suitable crystals (see A–Z Directory).
- Wear Black Tourmaline or Shungite constantly.
- Don't meditate or open yourself up psychically without considerable protection until the attack is over.
- Avoid drugs, alcohol or consciousness-altering substances.

Dealing with psychic attack from a known source

If you know where an attack is coming from, do not confront the person directly. Use your crystals to resolve the situation:

- Put yourself in a crystal bubble and wear Black Tourmaline or Shungite.

- If appropriate for you, invoke an angel of protection or any religious figure you find helpful.
- Disconnect from the person – remove yourself from their space and their energy – physically, emotionally, mentally and spiritually.
- Laugh about it to yourself, don't take it too seriously or give it too much energy.
- Take your attention away and turn it to something positive.
- Don't play their game or get pulled into power struggles.
- Don't see them, speak or think about them.
- Don't meditate or open yourself up psychically without appropriate protection.
- Avoid drugs, alcohol or consciousness-altering substances.
- If you have to, face up to them fearlessly with your boundaries strong.

201

(For further assistance see *Good Vibrations*.)

Hitchhikers 1: Thought forms

When one creates phantoms for oneself, one puts vampires into the world, and one must nourish these children of a voluntary nightmare with one's blood, one's life, one's intelligence, and one's reason, without ever satisfying them.

Eliphas Levi

A hitchhiker is something which attaches to your mind, your chakras or your auric field. This may be a discarnate being, something projected from an incarnate being, or a thought form. When you focus obsessively upon something, or have powerfully negative thoughts, it creates what is known as a thought form, or 'mind-made body'. Beneficial thought forms may also be created through repeated affirmations, intentions or incantations. In addition to being the product of your own mind, thought forms can arise from other people's perception or expectations of you, or from religious or other authoritarian dictates. Such forms may also arise from books or films or from your own imagination. Thought forms can also arise from those emails that people circulate that threaten you with dire consequences if they aren't sent on

– or promise rewards if they are. (Simply delete and send it out to the great cosmic recycling bin for disposal, then forget about it.)

Thought forms either lodge themselves in a chakra or the mental part of the auric field. Thought forms have been deliberately created by researchers.[4] External thought forms inhabit the lower astral realms – a place close to the earth plane where most spirits first pass after death of the body. They communicate through your chakras, sometimes appearing as an inner voice, sometimes as an external. External thought forms may appear to have separate and distinct life energy or they may be internalised. External thought forms are not necessarily beneficial although they may be. They may interfere in the lives of human beings by masquerading as a 'guide' (who spouts rubbish rather than sound guidance), or as a figure or inner voice that appears in quiet moments to offer guidance. Internal thought forms are usually experienced as a derogatory inner voice, or obsessive and potentially toxic thoughts that whirl around in your head.

Thought form

A 'mind-made body.' A thought form is a non-physical being generated by thought. It is usually experienced as a seemingly independent voice or thought that tries to control or influence behaviour from within your mind. It is generated by your own, or another person's, thoughts and beliefs. However, it may appear externally as an ethereal figure that may act as a guide or mentor.

The concept of a thought form was described by early members of the Theosophical movement, Annie Besant and CW Leadbeater, who said: "We have often heard it said that thoughts are things, and there are many among us who are persuaded of the truth of this statement. Yet very few of us have any clear idea as to what kind of thing a thought is…[5] Describing them as a "radiating vibration and a floating form", a concept that is recognizable in modern day quantum physics with its particle and wave formations, they placed thought forms into three categories:

An image of the thinker that could be sent to distant locations and perceived by sensitive others, even when the thinker has passed over.

An image of a material object associated with the thought – nowadays used in manifestation practices.

An independent image that expressed the inherent qualities of the thought. Low vibrational thoughts, such as anger, hate, lust, greed, and so on, would create thought forms that are dense in form and colour. Thoughts of a higher, more spiritual vibration would generate forms possessing a greater purity, clarity, and refinement.

Thought forms may be consciously directed toward anyone, but to be effective they must latch on to a similar vibration, feeling or thought in that person's aura. Or, find a weak spot or 'tear' in the aura. If they are unable to do so, they may well boomerang back on the sender.

How to recognize a negative thought form

- It doesn't *feel* or sound like it's your thought even though it's in your head.
- It doesn't have any connection with what you really want or who you are inside.
- It may resemble someone you know, especially if they have passed on.

- It gives you negative messages such as "that's a bad thing to do", "you're not good enough", "it's all your fault", "you'll never be/get what you want", "you don't deserve", "you're too clever for your own good".
- The guidance it gives is inappropriate and fallible.
- It *feels* subtly wrong.
- It seems to be stuck in a loop.
- It looks, talks or behaves exactly like a character from a film or book, especially a horror story.

- It has little substance or energy resonance to it, seeming more like a caricature or faded imprint.

Note: Such voices may, of course, be part of a mental disturbance that may require psychiatric treatment. If the methods given here do not work for you, it is wise to obtain medical assistance.

Dealing with thought forms

Internal thought forms can be quickly dissolved with a crystal supported by turning your thoughts around and affirming a positive viewpoint, or by recognizing the gift in a situation. Looking yourself in the eyes in a mirror and making a positive affirmation while holding a crystal is an excellent way to reprogram your mind – as is crystal EFT (see *Crystal Prescriptions volume 6*). If you are tormented by messages of how unlovely you are, for instance, you can say firmly, "I am lovable, I love myself, I am surrounded by love, I deserve love and I call love to me now" while tapping either side of your breastbone in the centre of your chest with a crystal.

It can be disconcerting to meet an external thought form while you are meditating or journeying – they have a nasty habit of leering in at you – and these thought forms need to be disposed of as quickly as possible. Laughing at them is an excellent weapon, as is simply ignoring them and shifting your focus to a higher vibration. An extremely useful tool for dealing with external thought forms is simply to point one of the thought clearing crystals at it and ask the crystal to remove it. If the thought form is internal, check which of the chakras would be the most appropriate for the crystal to work through. Aegerine is excellent for mental obsession or possession where you can't get someone out of your mind. Banded Agate removes a thought form projected by a guru or other authority figure. Remember to cleanse the crystals after use.

Hitchhikers 2: Ghosts and stuck spirits

Ghosts are subtle imprints left behind as a result of trauma or drama. Rather like a photograph or silent film, they endlessly replay their past, 'haunting' a place or constantly recreating a scene. They rarely hurt you, but they may frighten – and fear opens the way to difficulties. Fortunately it is easy to erase a ghostly imprint. Lost or stuck spirits are slightly different but can be dealt with in much the same way. They are usually souls who have passed to the other side too quickly or reluctantly, or who are held by unfinished business or unfulfilled desires. Sometimes all that is needed is for them to take a different view of the past, recognizing how things have changed – which may include the fact that they have died or time has moved on (see page 210). However, if the lost soul has become attached, stronger measures might be needed, and it may be necessary to seek expert assistance.

Ghostbusting

Petaltone Astral Clear placed on a clear Quartz crystal and left in place for a few hours dissolves the imprint. It also moves a lost or stuck spirit on to the light, as does a large Ametrine or Aventurine crystal appropriately dedicated.

Lost souls and stuck spirits

Some lost souls or stuck spirits may be deeply troubled and their interaction with the living may be malicious or they may be caught in an outdated viewpoint or intention. They may be members of your ancestral line who have become stuck because of a reluctance to move on. Stuck spirits may have unfinished business, or powerful desires especially for control over another person or to re-experience substance abuse. Or, they may not know how to move on or to let go. If you recognize the shift of perception or the turnaround required, they can see it through your eyes, releasing them. Sometimes these spirits do not even know that they are dead – after all, they feel very much alive! They may wonder why everyone around them appears to ignore them – and do all they can to gain attention. Working with seriously troubled or malicious souls is best left to an expert but it is possible to help lost souls to move on. This exercise works with a spirit or soul who is not directly attached to anyone but rather is free to wander.

If you are moving a stuck spirit on, always ask that it will be taken into the light and will find the guidance it needs. Compassion is a powerful tool in assisting such a being.

Moving on a stuck spirit

- Protect yourself before beginning. Wear a Black Tourmaline, Labradorite or other protective crystal and place yourself in a crystal bubble.
- Sit quietly and focus your attention on calling in higher helpers and guides to assist. Holding one of the crystals from the A–Z Directory, ask that the spirit be taken to the light by his or her guardian angel. This works well if the spirit has simply lost the way home. Petaltone Astral Clear or Clear Tone essences will assist the clearing. Sometimes simply recognizing that he or she is in the post-death state is all a spirit needs to move on of its own accord but you may need to do more.
- If you can communicate with the spirit, ask if there is anything you can do to assist, what he or she needs. The requests are usually simple and easy to arrange, and often relate to unfinished business. Once you have agreed to do or offer whatever is required, the spirit moves on. It may be that the spirit is still stuck in the viewpoint or purpose it had while he or she was alive. It may be necessary to check out with the spirit whether this purpose is still appropriate. Release may be achieved by

helping the spirit to take a different view by turning around to look at how things were in the past and how they have changed. (This is particularly so when a deceased relative is still 'protecting' a 'child' even though that child is now an adult.)

- If the spirit is deeply entrenched, or is still of the opinion that their advice and assistance is crucial for the well-being of someone still on Earth, calling in an expert is your best course of action, but do choose someone who moves them on to an appropriate place rather than just banishing them elsewhere to bother someone else. Your local spiritualist church, shamanic practitioner or metaphysical centre will be able to assist. In the meantime, keep your own energy high to ensure you are well protected.

Hitchhikers 3: Spirit attachment and undue influence

Spirit attachment is a more serious situation. It means that a discarnate spirit has entered or is affecting a living person's energy field. Undue influence is a lighter, more intermittent form of attachment that affects the auric field and the chakras. Attachment can only occur when an auric field or chakra is weak and depleted, and when you do not fully inhabit your body and your soul is not fully present so that an energetic 'gap' or vacuum is created. It often arises out of momentary loss of energy containment, 'loose boundaries', during high fever, drink or drug taking, or the effects of anaesthetic, shock or trauma. It is common in cases of depression or debilitating illnesses like ME, and may occasionally occur during sexual activity with a particularly predatory or spaced-out partner. Spirit attachment often occurs when a discarnate soul seeks to reconnect with a feeling or sensation that is missing in its new abode: alcohol, nicotine, caffeine and recreational drugs are just some such substances, but sex addiction is also common.

Spirit attachment can be seen in the eyes, which are

blank with 'no one home' most of the time, or 'someone else' looks out from them. The attaching spirit usually seeks to experience something it was addicted to in life, or to control or protect someone, or to feel safe. If the spirit is entrenched, it is a serious condition that needs experienced help and spirit release should not be attempted alone. However, if the spirit is lightly attached, crystals may assist.

Spirit attachment

Spirit attachment means that a, usually, discarnate spirit has entered a living person's energy field or is influencing it. However, it may be practised by someone who is still living and who has a specific agenda behind the 'possession' of another body. It can only occur when an auric field is weak and depleted, and when someone does not fully inhabit their body and the soul is not fully present so there is a 'gap' or vacuum. Grounding is the first step to dealing with the situation.

Signals that a spirit may be attached

The first four signs below are almost inevitably present in cases of spirit attachment or undue influence; others may be present intermittently. But please note, it is sensible to bear in mind that these signals may also be signs of a psychiatric illness or mental breakdown that may require additional treatment. Lost and malicious spirits are attracted to anyone who has no defences against them, so the more depressed or psychiatrically disturbed a person is, the more likely it is that there could be an attachment present. But equally, having an attachment may lead to mental or physical unrest.

- 'Blank' eyes
- Unable to make eye contact
- 'Someone else' looks out from the eyes
- Behaviour out of character with normal persona
- Obsessive or addictive behaviour including sexual
- Unusual thought patterns
- Intense dreams or fantasies with a nightmarish quality
- Hears voices
- A feeling of being controlled by someone else
- Sudden overwhelming bouts of tiredness or yawning
- Chronic fatigue, panic attacks, depression
- Overwhelming sugar cravings
- Person appears vague, nebulous and insubstantial
- Loss of libido or sudden exhaustion after physical contact

Signs that a spirit is trying to attach and protection is needed

Some of these signs are the same as already having a spirit attached, but there are some differences. Physical signs of a spirit attaching or trying to take over (you may feel this in your own body when working with someone else; check out if it's yours or theirs, it can become a useful signal to watch out for in future):

- feeling of heaviness/suffocation in limbs or chest
- palpitations
- anxiety attacks
- nausea or extreme weakness
- difficulty in breathing
- icy chills
- goose pimples
- dreadful smells
- body distortion or bruising
- cravings – especially drugs, nicotine, alcohol or sugar
- unease for no apparent reason

Attachments are not confined to human beings and may arise from thought forms or 'alien' sources. It is not always an external attachment *although it will feel like it is*. It may equally well be unwitting projection or repressed qualities or obsessive thoughts manifesting *apparently externally*. A spirit may also be attached to an object rather than a person. Not all attaching spirits will have left their physical body. The living can project themselves from the physical to 'possess' or overly influence the living. Attachments may arise from the thoughts and feelings of others who try to influence or control, or who try to clutch on to your energy field (keep your spleen chakra well protected). It is as though they have their hooks into you.

The advantage of using a crystal for this work is that it stands at the interface between you, the other person and the entity, creating a barrier so the entity does not attach to you after release. The crystal calls in angelic helpers and divine light and amplifies it, facilitating the work.

If you are inexperienced, or afraid, do not attempt to release a spirit yourself, seek professional help. (See also stuck souls, page 208.)

If you have had a spirit attachment yourself, pay special attention afterwards to healing your auric field, recreating your boundaries, and calling all the parts of your soul and your inner child home – which may need the assistance of an experienced practitioner or see *Crystal Prescriptions volume 6* and my *Book of Psychic Development* or *Good Vibrations*.

Attachments to the Chakras and Auric Field

Spirits may be attached through tears in the auric field or to a specific chakra (see page 135):

Typical attachments:
Gaia gateway: Energy leeches, control freaks, disembodied spirits seeking energy to remanifest or move on.

Earth star: Spirits of place, stuck spirits. If it is permanently open, you easily pick up negative energies from the ground or pick up 'spirits of place', either as attachments or as communication of events that have taken place.

Base and sacral: Previous partners, children, anyone you've ever had sex with, needy people, thought forms, unborn parents. Previous partners or significant others leave their imprint in these chakras and may continue to influence through the association.

Solar plexus: People with whom you have had an

emotional entanglement in the past whenever that may have been. Ancestral spirits, relatives, needy people. Invasion and energy leeching take place through this chakra. A 'stuck-open' solar plexus means you take on other people's feelings easily. You may well receive intuitions through your solar plexus as you unconsciously read other people's emotions.

Spleen: Psychic vampires, needy people, ex-partners. Psychic vampires leech your energy, as can past partners, children or parents, and hooks here are common.

Heart seed: Parts of your soul left in other lives or dimensions. If you have left parts of yourself at past life deaths or traumatic or deeply emotional experiences, then these parts may be attached and trying to influence you to complete unfinished business.

Heart: Anyone you have ever loved. Although it is difficult to imagine being possessed by those you have loved or who loved you, this chakra may be the site of a great many hooks. You may have given away parts of your heart and need to reclaim them (see page 188) or made promises that tie you to others (see page 179).

Higher heart: Guides, gurus or masters, mentors. Mentors, masters and gurus open the higher heart chakra, and in so doing tie you to them and not all masters or gurus have clean energy or the best of intentions.

Throat: Teachers, mentors, gurus, thought forms. A blocked throat chakra results in difficulty in communication – especially in not being able to speak your truth. Problems may arise from your own unvoiced intuitions and the dogmatic nature of a blocked throat chakra can leave you closed to intuitive solutions.

Brow: Thought forms, ancestors or relatives, lost souls. If the chakra is blocked, you cannot visualize or receive intuitions. You will be attached to the past, fearful and superstitious, and prone to create exactly what you fear most.

Soma: 'Lost souls', walk-ins. When this chakra is stuck open it is all too easy for spirits to attach. It can be used to detach the etheric body and help the soul move out.

Past life: Past life personas, soul fragments, thought forms from previous beliefs. If the chakras are stuck open, you will feel unsafe and overwhelmed by past life memories of trauma and violent death and fears, which leaves the way open for past life personas and thought forms to attach or remanifest.

Crown: Spiritual entities, lost souls, mentors. If it is stuck open, then you will be prey to illusions and false communicators as it leaves you open to thought forms, spirit attachment or undue influence.

Soul star: Ancestral spirits, ETs, 'lost souls'. Stuck open or blocked closed, it may lead to soul fragmentation, spirit attachment, ET invasion, or overwhelm by ancestral spirits.

Stellar gateway: So-called enlightened beings that are anything but. When it is stuck open, it may be a source of cosmic disinformation that leads to illusion, delusion, deception and disintegration that leaves you totally unable to function in the everyday world.

Causal vortex: Ancestors, thought forms, parts of the soul left in other incarnations.

Healing Spirit Attachment

The short method of detaching spirits given below can be very effective, but if you need further guidance see *Crystal Prescriptions volume 6*. As the attaching spirit is an uninvited guest and the influence unsought, it is not necessary to request another person's permission to assist them as the spirit is breaching their autonomy. You can do spirit detachment for yourself if you are aware of a spirit, but it is always wiser to seek experienced help who can deal with anything unexpected. However, the following is a useful emergency technique if someone else needs assistance. If the person is not present you can use their name or a photograph, or imagine them in the room with you. If you have strong energetic boundaries, you can also use yourself as a surrogate by performing the healing through your own body but this is not recommended unless you have previous experience of the technique.

To remove the attachment

- As soon as you begin, imagine throwing out an energetic net to trap the attaching spirit so that it cannot slip away. Do not pre-think the procedure before you begin or you will give the spirit warning and it may slip away.

- Lay out a crystal net at the start using Selenite, Bronzite or Black Tourmaline. This is particularly useful if you are working for someone who is not present, in which case lay the net over their name or a photograph. But keep your mind away from the reason until you have thrown the energetic net.
- Dowse each of the chakras in turn to ascertain where the spirit(s) is located. Be aware that there may be more than one.
- Place an appropriate spirit release crystal over the chakra and leave in place.
- Ask that the spirit will be directed to the light and picture the spirit, still in its net, being transported to the light where help awaits it.
- Check that there is no further attachment and close the chakra with an appropriate crystal.
- Check that the auric field is intact. Sweep all around it with Anandalite, Selenite or Flint to seal it, paying special attention to the earth star chakra.

It is essential when any kind of release has taken place that the aura be healed and sealed with Anandalite or other suitable crystal to prevent further incidents, and any crystals used are thoroughly cleansed.

The One-way Portal

To prevent the return of unwelcome guests when working with spirit release or banishing undesirable presences back to their own domain, lay a long Chlorite Quartz point down. Across it place a long Stibnite and over that a long Selenite to form an X. This one-way portal soaks up any negativity, releases a soul, thought form or entity, and sends it out of the earth plane and into light where it can be handled by wise mentors and soul-rescuers. It also returns 'alien' energies that have penetrated from elsewhere to their own place in or beyond the universes and blocks their return. But note that some 'alien presences' are actually internal projections that may need to be handled in a different way and may need the assistance of a qualified therapist.

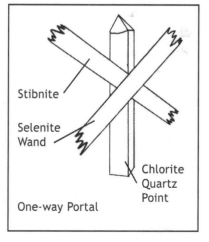

Stibnite

Selenite Wand

Chlorite Quartz Point

One-way Portal

Implants

Implants are subtly different to thought forms or undue influence, but they can be treated in the same way. Dowse to see where in the physical or energy body they are located and then proceed as per the previous page with appropriate crystals.

Hitchhikers 4: Attachment to objects including crystals

When I was little, I went to the Sahara desert and met an older woman with beautiful earrings that came all the way down to her stomach. She told me, "For us Tuareg, jewelry is not meant for decoration. It absorbs negative energy that comes your way." So think twice when you buy a vintage ring!
Sofia Boutella

It is not just people that may have spirits attached; objects can too *as may crystals and crystal skulls* – particularly where these have had cultic value. Jewellery, statues, fetishes, skulls and other objects may have a guardian spirit or a less desirable entity that may need to be released. In some cultures, jewellery is worn to absorb negative energy, as in the quote above, in exactly the same way as we wear a crystal to absorb or deflect negative vibes. The process of release is similar to attachments to the chakras. Bear in mind that:

- Letters or photographs may carry potentially toxic

emanations.

- Presents hold vibes – good or bad.
- Inherited items may not be energetically clean.
- Holiday souvenirs – or antiques – may have more attached than you bargained for as they carry an energetic history with them.
- Crystals may be holding negative energy when you acquire them.
- Crystal skulls do not always carry high mentor beings within them when first acquired.

Return, recycle or transform anything that is not conducive to your highest good.

If you suspect that an object is carrying ill wishing or an attachment of any kind, then it is wisest to dispose of it. But if you want to keep it, it will need thorough cleansing – and deprogramming if it is a crystal. If it is an item you

intend to get rid of, spray with Petaltone Astral Clear, Clear2Light or Z14 essence before parting with it, or burn it as this transmutes the energy. If it is an antique or an object with a cult or fetish connection, no matter how seemingly innocent, you may need to consult an appropriate practitioner to remove a former curse or intent.

Crystal hitchhikers

Crystals soaking up negative vibes is, in many cases, part of their job description. But, if not cleansed, they may get overstuffed and the negative energy starts to spill out again. They may also attract energetic beings from another dimension of being. Crystal skulls, in particular, have become much more common these days because of the wise mentors – allegedly – attached to them. Not all beings attached to crystals or skulls are necessarily of a higher, more aware vibration though. Do check them out thoroughly and don't assume anything. Remember, skulls hold both the oversoul of the type of crystal *and* a separate being from another dimension – or one from close to our own masquerading as a higher being. Just as people can pick up 'hitchhikers', spirits or beings that may not have the best of intentions and which draw on their energy, so too can crystals. Crystals do not necessarily hold vibes of sweetness and light. As we've already seen, until cleansed they hold the imprint of anyone who touched them. And not everyone has the best of intentions or the clearest of energies – which is why hitchhikers can transfer from person to crystal or skull – and on again. Some crystals may have attracted a hitchhiker that has far from benevolent intentions. The problem is that the dimension nearest to our own in vibration is the astral or etheric level. It's energetically dense and may be home to lost, mischievous or downright malevolent entities and con artists that are out to commit mayhem. They seek to influence for the worst and pass on disinformation. But there are others who are lost and simply trying to call attention to their plight in the same way that stuck souls may attach to a person. All very different to the crystal oversouls and mentors who inhabit a well tended crystal or skull. So never assume that, for instance, because you have bought a crystal skull it will have a high vibration being within it just as a high vibration crystal may have had its vibes brought low by what has attached to it. And a 'low' or earthy vibration crystal may equally well attract a mischievous being.

Blog extract: Crystals behaving badly

Someone recently asked on my Facebook page whether I'd noticed strange things happening around crystals. She'd found that, when she wore a particular Snowflake Obsidian donut, things started to go missing.

I'm used to the crystals themselves appearing and disappearing... But it seemed more likely that Snowflake Obsidian would make things visible. As I said in The Crystal Bible, *"it is a stone of purity providing balance for body, mind and spirit. Snowflake Obsidian helps you to recognize and release 'wrong thinking' and stressful mental patterns. It promotes dispassion and inner centring." Obsidian brings hidden imbalances up to the surface for transmutation, making the invisible visible. And the gentle 'snowflakes' help you to reach your higher self. So, Snowflake Obsidian is a great combination for deep self-examination and expanded awareness... [but behaving mischievously is not one of Snowflake Obsidian's qualities.]* www.judyhall.co.uk

If unwanted activity centres around a specific crystal or skull, or it becomes clear that the being attached to it does not have your highest good in mind, the first thing to do, as I recommended in the blog above, is give it a thorough cleanse and rededicate it to work for the highest good, as below. But more may be needed. You may, for instance, need to remove an unwanted entity from a crystal skull and replace it with a wiser being – if so follow the guidance for moving on a stuck spirit on page 210.

Cleansing a crystal skull, crystal or other object that carries a lower vibration entity

Giving your skull, crystal, or any suspect object, a thorough cleanse and saying firmly, "I direct that this being leave this skull [etc] and go to the light" may be sufficient to remove an unwanted presence. Or it may not. If the entity refuses to leave you may need a specialist essence to clear it out. Petaltone essence maker David Eastoe has several suitable potions and his contact details are in the Resources directory. If you work with the angels or other beings, ask for their assistance to remove the entity to a place where it receives help and healing. Do not merely banish it and leave it free to bother someone else.

- Place several drops of an essence such as Petaltone Z14 or Petaltone Astral Clear on the skull or crystal and ask that the presence be taken to the light or some suitable abode where it can no longer do mischief or pass on false information (use the one-way crystal portal on page 223 if appropriate).

- Place the skull or crystal in the sunlight for a thorough recharge before reactivating.

Reactivating a crystal skull

- Place your hands on either side of the skull and allow the crystal matrix to connect to you through the palm chakras (centre of each hand). When you are connected you have a sense that the skull is an extension of your awareness and you are an extension of the skull.
- Picture a beam of loving light going from your heart to the skull.
- Where possible, take it out into sunlight so that it is also activated by life-giving light.
- Once you are connected, tune into the energy in the skull at a higher level – take a deep breath and consciously lift your attention 'up' to the top of your head and beyond – moving your thumbs to the top of the cranium assists this process as does gently massaging the skull's third eye or crown chakra in a circular or figure-of-eight fashion.
- If the skull feels 'full', invite the being within it to awaken and make itself known to you.
- If the skull feels 'empty', invite the highest possible consciousness to enter the skull and communicate with you.
- The skull may offer you its name. If so greet it by name and welcome its presence into your life. If not, ask that this be given at an appropriate time.

- To close the connection to your skull, reverse the circular motion on the skull's third eye or crown chakra. Or simply place your hand over the skull's crown or third eye, and your other hand over your own.

Note: Crystal skulls may also be activated at expanded, multidimensional vibratory rates. This is advanced work and such activation is not covered here. [This material is extracted from *Crystal Skulls*; see this book for further information on working with crystal skulls.] However, your skull may spontaneously activate or have already been activated at these levels. If so, this becomes apparent in the information received and the energetic resonance of the skull.

And while we're on the subject of crystal skulls:

If you've bought a crystal skull and are wondering whether it carries the presence of a higher mentor being or a mischievous astral presence, ask yourself the following questions.

Checkpoint for successful crystal skull activation

- Are you hearing the communication, feeling or sensing it clearly?
- Is your skull communicating from the highest levels of awareness?
- Is your skull communication coherent?
- Is your skull speaking good sense?

- Does the energy of your skull *feel* good?
- Do you instinctively trust your skull?
- Is there a cognitive dissonance, a mismatch, between the inherent energies of the matrix of the skull itself and the consciousness that is trying to inhabit it?
- Does the energy of your skull feel jagged, disharmonious, 'off'?
- Is the communication garbled and disjointed? False?
- Do you feel worse rather than better when tuning into your skull or using it for healing?
- Is your skull telling you to do something you instinctively feel is wrong?
- Is your skull suggesting destructive actions?

If you answer yes to the first six points, congratulations, you have successfully activated your skull and connected to a higher consciousness mentor.

If you answer yes to the seventh question, it may be sensible to find a crystal skull in a material that is better suited to the type of consciousness that is trying to make contact. An earthy detoxifying healing-type crystal such as Smoky Quartz is not a comfortable home for a highly evolved, crystal mentor who wishes to channel wisdom for instance. A crystal matrix with an elevated vibration would be more suitable.

If you answer yes to the bottom five points, you may have inadvertently linked to a presence from the astral or lower etheric levels that requires ejecting or healing. A crystal skull itself may need further healing before commencing work. If so, see above.

Case History: An integrated approach

This case history shows the value of an integrated approach to psychic protection and illustrates the need to adapt and change as the situation moves through different stages. Fortunately the person concerned was very intuitive and had learned to trust that intuition. The first layout involved a Black Tourmaline and a 'bringing in light' Celtic Quartz grid, which brought things to the surface for a client who was experiencing problems within her family. She had been feeling as though she was under severe psychic attack and needed to keep her energies clear in order to deal with the family member in question. It was ongoing work as my client reported:

The grid is bringing in great results. I supplemented it as after I did the grid with your crystals I got an email from the family member in question which was unpleasant. I felt bullied after this email.

I did reply to the email factually giving feedback that I understood that the issues underneath their recent behaviours were as a result of their emotional anxiety. Whereas I understood, I had a responsibility to not cave-in and had to show tough love.

But I was upset by the email and the attack so I did another separate grid for bullying.

So I put Quartz at the top. Then Black Tourmaline and initially a skull which I thought was Snowflake Obsidian underneath followed by a Bloodstone and a Citrine. The energy felt wrong and sticky.

So I googled your advice on Snowflake Obsidian. I was surprised at the serendipity – you had written on this in a blog and in the same breath about hitchhikers on skulls. On further examination I saw the skull purchased on Amazon was actually Dalmatian Stone and wrongly described on my purchase!!

However, I did the process you recommended to clear the skull and immediately it felt clear. I wrapped the skull away and put in a purple cloth for later.

I replaced the place in the grid with a Red Jasper dragon. It felt good!

After this everything changed; so far it is going in the right direction with the family member and I got pleasant texts and messages – in a loving tone. We have arranged to meet later on.

I will do your karmic workshop in February at the College of Psychic studies and bring the skull in case anyone wants to work on it but I am minded to throw it away!!!

It will take time my healing with the family member, but I realise I have to do this work and [have been] given the opportunity to do it.

When she brought the Dalmatian skull to the workshop we cleansed it and put it in the ancestral karmic clearing grid for a short time (see *Crystal Prescriptions volume 6*). We then cleansed it again and called in a higher being to the skull. My client offered it to workshop participants to assist anyone who had a child that needed help and that offer was gratefully accepted. More work on the family problem has followed and further assistance has become available through a series of serendipitous synchronicities.

The Uncursing Ritual

Curses, whether personal or transgenerational, can leave you vulnerable to psychic invasion or attack as the blight continues through time until the core energy is dissolved. You may have become inadvertently – and unconsciously – caught up in a karmic or transgenerational curse (see *Crystal Prescriptions volume 6*). This ritual is excellent for removing past life curses that hold a soul part in thrall but it also clears ancestral curses and attachments, thought forms and entities that could be making you vulnerable at a subtle level. You can do it for yourself or on another person.

- Place four Tourmalinated Quartz or Black Tourmalines at each corner of a rectangle large enough to lie down in (using a cloth to outline the space is helpful). Join the crystals up with a wand to create a sacred space into which you can step or place the person you are working on. The ritual is best conducted lying down.

- Place a fifth Tourmalinated Quartz or Black Tourmaline crystal just below the breastbone above the solar plexus. Hold a Nuummite crystal in your right hand (a wand or wedge shape is ideal) and a Novaculite or Flint shard in your left hand (other uncursing crystals will be found in the A–Z Directory).

- Beginning above the crown chakra, place both hands above the head and 'comb' across the chakra about a hand's breadth above the body with each of the crystals in turn, starting with the Novaculite (be careful as this flinty crystal can be very sharp). As you work on the chakra, ask that you or the person you are working on and all the ancestral line be released from all and any curses/thought forms that have been put at any time in the past.

- Moving your hands in a figure of eight formation that crosses and then moves apart again at each chakra, move down the body cleansing and clearing each chakra in turn.

- When you reach the base chakra, work back up the chakras again with the same sweeping figure of eight movement until you reach the crown. Continue until the chakras feel clear.

- Now close your eyes and ask that the person who placed the curse will make him or herself known to you. You may see a clear picture or get a prickling sensation on one side of your head or a pain somewhere in your body – in which case move the Tourmalinated Quartz over the spot either on your own body or that of your patient to absorb the pain. Talk to this person, discuss why the curse was placed, how it can be removed and what reparation, if any, is required on either side. Offer and accept forgiveness. Then ask that the curse be lifted from the recipient and all the generations to come and those who have gone before, everyone who has been affected. Feel the effect of the crystals radiating back through time and forward into the future freed from the effects of the curse and bringing beneficial experiences and joyful learning to everyone involved.

- Work through each chakra again in turn with the Novaculite and Nuummite, again healing and sealing each one with light.
- Find a place where you can set out the Tourmalinated grid and leave it to continue its work.

Technological Incompatibility

If you experience constant computer crashes and the like, your auric field might well be incompatible with technology, particularly if you are highly intuitive or under ill wishing (see page 197). You may notice that when you are having a particularly 'bad computer day' and become more and more stressed, the machine responds in kind. The computer is interacting with your energy. It feels like it is being energetically attacked and so responds accordingly. Screening the computer from your energies may sometimes be appropriate in addition to screening you from the computer (see *Crystal Prescriptions volume 3*). This is so especially if you are ungrounded and not well anchored in everyday reality. Some people have a strong personal magnetic field to which technology may react adversely. But electrical equipment is particularly sensitive to subtle vibrations and so a ghost in the machine can be a reality. Computers also respond adversely to the presence of ghosts and disembodied spirits in the environment. If you suspect that this is the case, take appropriate action to move them on.

Crystal Solution: Wear small stones or place large ones between yourself and the computer but remember to cleanse regularly. Try:

• Fluorite, Smoky Quartz, Shungite, Lepidolite (see A–Z Directory).

Travel Safely

Travelling may take you into a negative environment, especially if you are jammed alongside other people who are full of fear or anger or other negative emotions, or just exhausted themselves. It can be all too easy to absorb their thoughts and feelings – and they can leech your energy even where you are, apparently, protected by your car. With the constant threat of terrorist activity (or so we are constantly told), many people are frightened to travel at all and you may need to take control of your life in order not to be manipulated or affected by it. Remember that being afraid is likely to attract exactly what you fear, whilst remaining calm and unfazed enhances your chances of a safe journey. But you may also need to consider that a car or a plane is a cage that does not allow electromagnetic frequencies to dissipate. And, in most planes, the 'air' is actually recycled from the engines and so contains petro-chemical pollutants. If you are electro- or chemically-sensitive you need to take the same precautions as you would within your home or work environment (see pages 69 and 72). Taking the right precautions before you travel helps you to arrive fresh and unscathed (see Travel protection crystals in the A–Z Directory).

Your car

Your car is essentially a metal cage that encloses you in an EMF field so if you are electro- or chemically-sensitive, you need to take steps to discharge the static field and protect yourself. Shungite around your neck, between the seats or on your dashboard assists, as does putting pieces into the door pockets so that you are enclosed in a Shungite net. Blue Chalcedony keeps you protected and Preseli Bluestone on your keyring not only protects you but also enhances your sense of direction.

Road rage is on the increase, which may be due in part to the proliferation of EMF fields in modern cars. To protect yourself against this, keep a Carnelian in your car. The gentle pink variety is ideal. Eye of the Storm (Judy's Jasper) helps you to keep calm at all times and Rhodonite manages anger.

Public transport

If you become depleted when travelling in the company of other people:

- Wear a Black Tourmaline to block energies or a Labradorite crystal around your neck to screen your energies. (Cleanse after use as crystals will quickly absorb 'bad vibes'.)
- Cross your ankles and your wrists – this seals your energy circuit.

Planes also act as EMF cages and may drastically affect

your energy. If you have a long flight:

- Keep a piece of Preseli Bluestone in your pocket or over your heart chakra to travel safely and avoid jet lag.

If you are in a high crime area, wear Sardonyx. Turquoise is a very old amulet stone used for protection while on land, and Aquamarine for travels on the sea.

Stealth journeys

It you want to travel without attracting unwanted attention:

- Wear Snakeskin or Leopardskin Agate or Nuummite, or hold a Desert Rose.

This works for shamanic or more pragmatic journeying in areas where you do not want to attract attention.

Amulets

The splendid stones! The splendid stones! The stones of abundance and of joy.

Made resplendent for the flesh of the gods. The hulalini stone, the sirgarru stone, the hulalu stone (Pearl), the andu stone, the uknu (Lapis Lazuli) stone. The dushu stone, the precious stone elmeshu (Diamond/Quartz), perfect in celestial beauty.

The stone of the pingu is set in gold. Placed upon the shining breast of the king as an ornament. Azagsud, high-priest of Bel, make them shine, make them sparkle!

Let the evil one keep aloof from the dwelling!

La Magie Assyrienne, translation by Fossey, 1902

This Assyrian text is an incantation spoken while creating an amulet with seven crystals to protect the breast of the king and form a fitting home for the gods. It is likely that the stones involved were connected to the visible planets and the luminaries but translation difficulties make it impossible to be sure. Amulets were dedicated to the gods and the gods were linked to the planets. The Romans, ancient Greeks and Egyptians made similar astrological connections. An amulet called in the protection of the god. Such protective amulets have been used since time immemorial but amulets may also be used to attract good fortune and the 'favour of the gods'.

The world has no greater thing; if any one have this with him he will be given whatever he asks for; it also assuages the wrath of kings and despots, and whatever the wearer says will be believed. Whoever bears this stone, which is a gem, and pronounces the name engraved upon it, will find all doors open, while bonds and stone walls will be rent asunder.

The Leyden Papyrus (3rd century CE)

The quotation above is taken from the archaic traditions of Egypt. The stone referred to is usually translated as Bloodstone but not as we in the modern world know that stone. Rather it is Hematite, which was strongly associated with blood because of its raw red colour. Hematite was universally regarded as magical because, with polishing, it became transformed into a silvery colour. It is just one of the many examples of the uses of amulets taken from the magical papyri of Egypt. As may be seen from the quotation, amulets were not only protective, they also 'opened doors'.

As the writer George Kunz, a specialist in the history of crystal usage, explained:

One of the special uses of amulets was for seafaring people, for, in ancient times especially, all who went down to the sea in ships were greatly in need of protection from the fury of the elements when they embarked in their small sailing-vessels. A fragment of a Greek Lapidary, 15 probably written in the third or fourth century of our era, gives a list of seven amulets peculiarly adapted for this purpose. The number might suggest a connection with the days of the week, and the amulets were perhaps regarded as most efficacious when used on the respective days.

In the first were set a carbuncle [Garnet] and a chalcedony; this amulet protected sailors from drowning. The second had for its gem either of two varieties of the adamas [Quartz], one, the Macedonian, being likened to ice (this was probably rock-crystal), while the other, the Indian, of a silvery hue, may possibly have been our corundum [Ruby or Sapphire]; however, the Macedonian stone was regarded as the better. The third amulet bore the beryl, "transparent, brilliant, and of a sea-green hue," evidently the aquamarine beryl; this banished fear. The fourth had for its gem the druops, "white in the centre," probably the variety of agate so much favored as a protector against the spell of the Evil Eye. A coral was placed in the fifth amulet, and this was to be attached to the prow of the ship with strips of seal-skin; it guarded the vessel from winds and waves in all waters. For the sixth amulet the ophiokiolus stone was selected, most probably a kind of banded agate, for it is said to have been girdled with stripes like the body of a snake; whoever wore this had no need to fear the surging ocean. The seventh and last of these nautical amulets bore a stone called opsianos, apparently a resinous or bituminous material, possibly a kind of jet; this came from Phrygia and Galatia, and the amulet wherein it was set was a great protection for all who journeyed by sea or by river.

A gemstone amulet list

Whosoever owns the true turquoise set in gold will not injure any of his limbs when he falls, whether he be riding or walking, so long as he has the stone with him.
Steinbuch [13th century German stonebook]

The following list incorporates both traditional and modern stones:

Agate: Traditionally protects against danger, worldly troubles, harmful spirits and whilst travelling.

Amber: Aura protector.

Amethyst: Traditionally worn to protect against drunkenness, hailstorms, thunderstorms and lightning, witchcraft and psychic attack. Protecting while travelling, it was believed to protect soldiers from harm. Foils attempts by others to steal your power.

Angelite: Calls in angelic protection.

Apache Tear: Aura protection and a shield against environmental stresses.

Aquamarine: Traditional protection against drowning, worn when travelling over water. Said by Kunz to counteract "the lure of dark spirits and procure wise ones".

Beryl: Protection in battle or against litigation.

Black Onyx: Protects from harmful spirits and environmental stresses. Blocks negative influences.

Black Tourmaline: Creates a psychic shield against outside influences such as psychic attack, psychic vampires, spirit possession, thought forms and harmful spirit intrusions. Protects against spells, ill wishing, microwaves, radiation, and environmental and geopathic stresses.

Bloodstone: Guards against deception. Protects against harmful spirits, wounds and insect bites. Used in ancient times to ensure the health of babies and children.

Blue Topaz: Protects from harm.

Carnelian: Traditionally said to shield against the powers of the devil and harmful spirits. Used in ancient times to protect young children. Traditionally safeguards against injury caused by falling walls or buildings.

Chalcedony: Protection against nightmares and 'phantoms of the night'.

Chrysoberyl: Charm against evil spirits.

Chrysoprase: Protection against hanging.

Citrine: Attracts good fortune and makes you less susceptible to negative influences.

Diamond: Protects against plague and pestilence and inconstancy on the part of a partner.

Emerald: Keeps away evil spirits and shields against the powers of magicians. Ensures constancy in a relationship.

Epidote: Protects during challenging circumstances.

Eye Agate/Cat's Eye: Wards off the evil eye.

Fluorite: Psychic shield. Protects against computer and EMF stress.

Garnet: Protection against bullet wounds.

Jade: Protects children from childhood diseases and the spleen chakra from vampirisation.

Jasper: Protection against the bite of venomous creatures and harmful spirits.

Jet: Screens out negative energy.

Labradorite: Screens out negative energy. Protects against psychic attack, psychic vampirism, negative alien interference and implants, negative attachments, and spirit possession.

Lapis Lazuli: Protection in the underworld.

Lodestone: Protection against seduction by a beautiful woman. Alexander the Great is said to have provided his soldiers with Lodestone amulets to protect them from djinns, "enchantments and all the machinations of malignant spirits".

Malachite: Protects against radiation, poisoning and psychic attack. Traditionally used to protect children from evil spirits and adults from enchantments.

Marcasite: Shields from negative energy and entities.

Moonstone: Protects while travelling on water.

Obsidian: Blocks negative influences and toxic environmental energies.

Opal: Guards against ill wishers.

Peridot: Shield for the body against negative forces and jealousy, and protection against night terrors.

Quartz: Powerfully protective on all levels.

Ruby: Traditionally shields against psychic attack or bullet wounds and protects against misfortune.

Sapphire: Traditionally used as an antidote or protection against poisoning and also to guard against fraud.

Sard: Traditionally created, a screen against incantations and sorcery.

Serpentine: Protected against venomous bites.

Smoky Quartz: Acts as a buffer against harm and negative influences.

Star Sapphire: Traditionally guards against the evil eye.

Sugilite: Protects the soul from shocks and disappointments.

Tiger's Eye: Protects against spirit attachment. Protects whilst travelling in cars.

Turquoise: Protects against physical injury, especially broken bones, and from danger. Traditionally used as an amulet when horse riding.

Zircon: Traditionally guards against being struck by lightning or struck down by pestilence.

Creating your own amulet

- Select a suitable stone from the A–Z Directory or the list above.
- Cleanse it thoroughly.
- Hold the stone in your hands and ask that it will protect you (or whatever your intention is for the amulet).
- Keep it about your person constantly.
- Whenever you feel anxious or threatened, touch the amulet to remind yourself that you are protected.

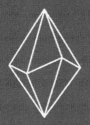

Part IV
A-Z Directory

Using this directory

In this directory you will find an A–Z list of issues that contribute to the need for space clearing or psychic protection with their appropriate healing stones in addition to Feng Shui stones. Most entries have several crystals listed that would be beneficial. There is a choice because everyone, and every environment, is subtly different. Crystals work holistically acting at a causal level on the whole person or the environment. You will need to find the protection that interacts best with your specific vibrations. Similarly, what needs clearing in one home may be very different to another that is experiencing similar difficulties but from a different cause. So, different crystals and grids will be appropriate. Many of the entries have a chakra or chakras associated with them. This means that the issue can be treated through putting appropriate stones on the chakra and leaving in place for 15–20 minutes or so. Or, the crystal can be placed in the environment or on a map – dowse for its precise position.

Occasionally certain crystals are contraindicated and you will find these listed in the directory under Contraindications (page 275).

To ascertain the best crystal for you

To ascertain which crystal will be most beneficial for you or for your purpose, follow the dowsing directions on page 16. Hold the pendulum in your most receptive hand. Put the forefinger of your other hand on the condition or issue in the directory. Slowly run your finger along the list of possible crystals, noting whether you get a 'yes' or 'no' response. Check the whole list to see which 'yes' response is strongest as there may well be two or three that would be appropriate, or you may need to use several crystals in combination. Another way to do this, if you have several of the crystals available, is to touch each crystal in turn, again noting the 'yes' or 'no' response – open your palm chakras before doing so (see page 19).

If you get a no response when checking out a condition or site, open your palm chakras, touch each of the capital letters in turn dowsing until you receive a yes, then run your finger down the conditions. This may well reveal something that underlies the apparent issue. If you get no response at all, it may be that you need to remove yourself from a geopathically stressed place, or that the question should be asked at another time.

Alternatively, use your intuition or open the palm chakras in your hands and allow your hands to simply find the right crystal, without thinking about it, which will feel tingly or may jump out of your hands as you pick it up.

– A –

Abuse: Apricot Quartz, Azeztulite with Morganite, Eilat Stone, Golden Healer, Honey Opal, Lazurine, Lemurian Jade, Morganite, Pink Crackle Quartz, Proustite, Red Quartz, Rhodonite, Rose Quartz, Septarian, Shiva Lingam, Smoky Amethyst, Smoky Citrine, Xenotine. *Chakra:* base, sacral, three-chambered heart, causal vortex

  break away from: Cradle of Humankind, Freedom Stone, Xenotine. *Chakra:* sacral and solar plexus

  clear emotional: Apricot Quartz, Azeztulite with Morganite, Cradle of Humankind, Honey Opal, Lazurine, Mount Shasta Opal, Rosophia, Smoky Rose Quartz, Tugtupite, Xenotine. *Chakra:* sacral, heart

  sexual, heal: Apricot Quartz, Eilat Stone, Golden Healer, Proustite, Shiva Lingam. *Chakra:* base, sacral

Acceptance of physical body: Celestobarite, Cradle of Humankind, Empowerite, Golden Healer, Keyiapo, Llanite (Llanoite), Riebekite with Sugilite and Bustamite, Schalenblende, Thompsonite and see Incarnation page 306. *Chakra:* earth star, base, dantien, crown

Addiction, understand causes of: Auralite 23, Carnelian, Crystal Cap Amethyst, Fenster Quartz, Iolite, Kornerupine, Malachite, Red Amethyst, Rose Quartz, Smoky Amethyst, Vera Cruz Amethyst. *Chakra:* past life, base, causal vortex

Addictions: Amethyst, Amethyst Elestial Quartz, Aventurine, Azurite, Banded Agate, Black Tourmaline, Blue Fluorite, Botswana Agate, Brandenberg Amethyst,

Carnelian, Celestite, Citrine, Crackled Fire Agate, Danburite, Fenster Quartz, Golden Selenite, Green Tourmaline, Iolite, Lazulite, Lepidolite, Peridot, Quartz, Selenite, Smoky Amethyst, Smoky Quartz, Tantalite, Vera Cruz. *Chakra:* base, sacral, dantien (or take as alcohol-free essence or carry at all times)

Adverse environmental factors: Amazonite, Aragonite, Black Tourmaline, Champagne Aura Quartz, Chlorite Quartz, Diamond, Ethiopian Opal, Eye of the Storm, Fulgarite, Galena (wash hands after use, make essence by indirect method), Granite, Graphite, Heulandite, Khutnohorite, Marble, Natrolite, Orgonite, Petrified Wood, Pollucite, Preseli Bluestone, Rose Quartz, Scolecite, Selenite, Shieldite, Shiva Lingam, Shungite, Smoky Amethyst, Smoky Elestial Quartz, Smoky Quartz, Stilbite, Thompsonite, Trummer Jasper. *Chakra:* earth star, dantien. Place crystal at four corners of house or site, on computer etc.

Akashic Record, read: Afghanite, Amphibole, Ancestralite, Andescine Labradorite, Blue Aventurine, Blue Euclase, Brandenberg Amethyst, Brookite, Cathedral Quartz, Celestial Quartz, Celestobarite, Chinese Writing Quartz, Chrysotile, Cradle of Humankind, Dumortierite, Eilat Stone, Heulandite, Keyiapo, Lemurian Aquitane Calcite, Merkabite Calcite, Merlinite, Optical Calcite, Phosphosiderite, Prehnite, Prophecy Stone, Serpentine in Obsidian, Sichuan Quartz, Tanzanite, Tibetan Black Spot Quartz, Tremolite, Trigonic Quartz. *Chakra:* past life, third eye, crown, causal vortex

Align self with spiritual energy: Anandalite, Andean Blue Opal, Annabergite, Celadonite, Ethiopian Opal, Prophecy Stone, Ruby Lavender Quartz, Sillimanite. *Chakra:* crown, soul star, stellar gateway

Align soul with physical body: Ajo Blue Calcite, Anandalite™, Cradle of Humankind, Empowerite, Larvikite, Schalenblende, Scheelite, Scolecite, Sichuan Quartz, Sillimanite, Thompsonite. Hold over head or solar plexus.

Alta major chakra: Afghanite, African Jade (Budd Stone), Anandalite, Andara Glass, Angelinite, Angel's Wing Calcite, Apatite, Auralite 23, Aurichalcite, Azeztulite, Black Moonstone, Blue Kyanite, Blue Moonstone, Brandenberg Amethyst, Budd Stone (African Jade), Cradle of Humankind, Crystal Cap Amethyst, Diaspore (Zultanite), Emerald, Ethiopian Opal, Eye of the Storm (Judy's Jasper), Fire and Ice Quartz, Fluorapatite, Garnet in Pyroxene, Golden Healer, Golden Herkimer Diamond, Graphic Smoky Quartz, Green Ridge Quartz, Herkimer Diamond, Holly Agate, Hungarian Quartz, Petalite, Phenacite, Preseli Bluestone, Rainbow Covellite, Rainbow Mayanite, Red Agate, Red Amethyst, Rosophia. Place at base of skull.

> **balance and align:** Anandalite, Brandenberg Amethyst, Crystal Cap Amethyst, Green Ridge Quartz, Preseli Bluestone on soma chakra with Angel's Wing Calcite, Blue Kyanite or Herkimer Diamond on base of skull
>
> **spin too rapid/stuck open:** African Jade (Budd Stone),

Auralite 23, Black Moonstone, Calcite, Eye of the Storm, Flint, Golden Healer, Graphic Smoky Quartz

spin too sluggish/stuck closed: Blue Moonstone, Diaspore, Ethiopian Opal, Herkimer Diamond, Quartz, Red Agate

Ancestral issues: Ancestralite, Celtic Quartz, Cradle of Humankind, Golden Healer, Lakelandite, Porphyrite (Chinese Letter Stone). *Chakra:* past life, causal vortex, alta major

Ancestral line, healing: Amber, Ancestralite, Brandenberg Amethyst, Candle Quartz, Chlorite Quartz, Cradle of Humankind, Crinoidal Limestone, Datolite, Fairy Quartz, Golden Healer, Ilmenite, Kambaba Jasper, Lemurian Aquitane Calcite, Mohawkite, Prasiolite, Preserved Wood, Rainforest Jasper, Shaman Quartz, Smoky Elestial Quartz, Spirit Quartz, Stromatolite. *Chakra:* past life, base, causal vortex

Ancestral patterns: Ancestralite, Anthrophyllite, Arfvedsonite, Candle Quartz, Celadonite, Celtic Quartz, Cradle of Humankind, Crinoidal Limestone, Eclipse Stone, Garnet in Quartz, Glendonite, Golden Healer, Green Ridge Quartz, Holly Agate, Lakelandite, Mohawkite, Porphyrite (Chinese Letter Stone), Prasiolite, Rainbow Covellite, Rainbow Mayanite, Scheelite, Shaman Quartz with Chlorite, Starseed Quartz. *Chakra:* past life, causal vortex, alta major

Angelic protection, invoke: Angelite, Angel's Wing Calcite, Celestite, Selenite, Seraphinite

Anger, ameliorate: Cinnabar in Jasper, Ethiopian Opal,

Nzuri Moyo, Rhodonite. *Chakra:* base, dantien

Antibacterial and antiviral: Amber, Anhydrite, Blue Euclase, Blue Tourmaline (Indicolite), Cathedral Quartz, Golden Healer Quartz, Green Calcite, Honey Opal, Iolite, Malachite, Owyhee Blue Opal, Proustite, Quantum Quattro, Que Sera, Shungite, Sulphur, Sulphur in Quartz, Trummer Jasper, Wonder Stone. Bathe in crystal essence, drink Shungite activated water or apply stone over site.

Antisocial behaviour/aggression: Amethyst, Blizzard Stone, Bloodstone, Carnelian, Eye of the Storm, Freedom Stone, Rose Quartz, Ruby, Sardonyx, Selenite, Shungite, Sodalite. Place in environment.

Antistatic: Amber, Fire Agate, Lepidolite, Quartz, Rose Quartz, Shungite, Sodalite, Tourmaline

Anxiety: Amber, Amethyst, Aventurine, Chrysoprase, Emerald, Eye of the Storm, Galaxyite, Green Calcite, Hematite, Khutnohorite, Kunzite, Labradorite, Lemurian Aquitane Calcite, Lemurian Gold Opal, Moonstone, Nzuri Moyo, Oceanite, Owyhee Blue Opal, Pyrite, Pyrite in Magnesite, Riebekite with Sugilite and Bustamite, Rose Quartz, Rutilated Quartz, Scolecite, Smithsonite, Strawberry Quartz, Tanzanite, Thunder Egg, Tiger's Eye, Tourmaline, Tremolite, Tugtupite. *Chakra:* earth star, base, solar plexus

Assimilate change: Actinolite, Basalt, Bismuth, Blue Euclase, Brandenberg Amethyst, Clevelandite, Conichalcite, Cradle of Humankind, Frondellite, Green Ridge Quartz, Luxullianite, Nunderite, Nuummite, Shift Crystal, Tangerose. *Chakra:* three-chambered heart

Astral travel, protection during: Amethyst, Brecciated Jasper, Condor Agate, Eye of the Storm, Kyanite, Red Jasper, Snakeskin Agate, Stibnite, Yellow Jasper. *Chakra:* soma

Atmospheric pollutants, remove: Amber, Black Tourmaline, Chlorite Quartz, Diamond, Elestial Quartz, Fulgarite, Graphite, Halite, Hanksite, Heulandite, Natrolite, Nuummite, Orgonite, Paraiba Tourmaline, Pollucite, Pyrite and Sphalerite, Quantum Quattro, Scolecite, Shaman Quartz, Shieldite, Shungite, Smoky Quartz, Sodalite, Stilbite, Thompsonite, Turquoise. *Chakra:* earth star. Or place in environment.

Attachment, recognize and detach: Brandenberg, Charoite, Cradle of Humankind, Drusy Golden Healer, Hemimorphite, Lemurian Seed, Pink Crackle Quartz, Rainbow Mayanite, Tinguaite. *Chakra:* as appropriate.

Attachments, remove: Celtic Quartz, Charoite, Drusy Golden Healer, Flint, Ilmenite, Jasper, Larvikite, Lemurian Seed, Rainbow Mayanite, Shungite, Smoky Amethyst, Stibnite, Tantalite, Tinguaite, and see Spirit release page 336. *Chakra:* or site as appropriate

Attitude, change: Amethyst Spirit Quartz, Axinite, Dream Quartz, Drusy Danburite, Eclipse Stone, Fluorapatite, Heulandite, Lilac Crackle Quartz, Luxullianite, Purpurite, Satyaloka Quartz, Smoky Citrine, Stichtite, Wavellite

Aura, negative patterns embedded in, dissolve: Amechlorite, Amphibole Quartz, Anandalite, Ancestralite, Arfvedsonite, Bronzite, Cradle of

Humankind, Dumortierite, Flint, Garnet in Quartz, Glendonite, Golden Healer, Lakelandite, Nuummite with Novaculite, Rainbow Covellite, Rainbow Mayanite, Scheelite, Spectrolite, Tantalite. 'Comb' over aura.

Aura, protect: Amber, Amethyst, Anandalite, Beryllonite, Black Tourmaline, Eye of the Storm, Fire Agate, Golden Healer, Hackmanite, Honey Phantom Calcite, Labradorite, Mahogany Sheen Obsidian, Master Shamanite, Mohawkite, Nunderite, Paraiba Tourmaline, Polychrome Jasper, Scolecite, Sunstone, Tantalite, Tiger's Eye. *Chakra:* higher heart. Or wear continuously, hold in front of solar plexus or sweep aura.

Aura, seal: Actinolite, Anandalite, Andean Blue Opal, Brookite, Eye of the Storm, Feather Pyrite, Fire Agate, Galaxyite, Golden Healer, Honey Phantom Calcite, Labradorite, Lorenzenite (Ramsayite), Molybdenite in Quartz, Nunderite, Pyromorphite, Serpentine in Obsidian, Smoky Amethyst, Spectrolite, Tantalite, Thunder Egg, Tiger's Eye, Valentinite and Stibnite, Xenotine

Aura, stabilize: Ajo Blue Calcite, Anandalite, Brookite, Ethiopian Opal, Flint, Golden Healer, Granite, Mtrolite, Poppy Jasper, Tantalite, Thunder Egg. *Chakra:* earth star

Auric blockages, remove: Ajo Quartz, Arfvedsonite, Beryllonite, Cradle of Humankind, Fire and Ice Quartz, Flint, Golden Healer, Green Aventurine, Labradorite, Lemurian Seed, Prehnite with Epidote, Rainbow Mayanite, Rhodozite, Serpentine in Obsidian, Strawberry Lemurian. Circle over site.

Auric cleansing: Amber, Amechlorite, Amethyst, Ametrine, Anandalite, Black Kyanite, Brown Jasper, Calcite, Citrine Spirit Quartz, Dravite Tourmaline, Fire and Ice Quartz, Flint, Frondellite with Strengite, Golden Healer, Green Jasper, Herkimer Diamond, Holly Agate, Keyiapo, Lemurian Seed Quartz, Lepidocrosite, Mystic Topaz, Nuummite, Phlogopite, Pumice, Pyrite in Quartz, Pyrite and Sphalerite, Quartz, Rainbow Mayanite, Rainbow Obsidian, Rutile, Smoky Quartz, Tourmaline. 'Comb' aura thoroughly.

Auric cords, remove: Amechlorite, Flint, Lemurian Aquitane Calcite, Lemurian Seed, Nunderite, Nuummite with Novaculite, Rainbow Mayanite. Circle over site.

Auric energy leakage, guard against: Eudialyte, Eye of the Storm, Fire Agate, Gaspeite, Labradorite, Pyrite in Quartz, Quartz with Mica, Spectrolite. *Chakra:* higher heart. Wear constantly.

Auric entities, remove: Amechlorite, Drusy Golden Healer, Flint, Frondellite plus Strengite, Keyiapo, Klinoptilolith, Larvikite, Pyromorphite, Rainbow Mayanite, Selenite Phantom, and see Entities page 292. *Chakra:* base, sacral, solar plexus, spleen, third eye

Auric 'holes'/breaks: Aegerine, Anandalite, Brookite, Chinese Red Quartz, Eye of the Storm, Fire Agate, Green Ridge Quartz, Labradorite, Lemurian Seed, Scolecite. Place over site.

Auric implants/mental attachments, remove: Amechlorite, Anandalite, Chinese Red Quartz, Cradle of Humankind, Cryolite, Drusy Golden Healer, Flint,

Frondellite with Strengite, Holly Agate, Ilmenite, Klinoptilolith, Lemurian Aquitane Calcite, Lemurian Seed, Molybdenite in Quartz, Rainbow Mayanite, Tantalite, Tinguaite. *Chakra:* third eye. Place on chakra until released, then purify stone immediately.

Authority figures, difficulties with: Ancestralite, Barite, Cradle of Humankind, Freedom Stone, Lakelandite, Pietersite, Pyrophyllite, Sceptre Quartz, Sonora Sunrise. *Chakra:* dantien

Autonomy: Candle Quartz, Cradle of Humankind, Faden Quartz, Flint, Freedom Stone, Frondellite with Strengite, Pietersite, Pyrolusite, Pyrophyllite, Rhodolite Garnet, Ussingite. *Chakra:* dantien

Baggage, release emotional: Chrysotile in Serpentine, Cumberlandite, Eclipse Stone, Garnet in Quartz, Graphic Smoky Quartz (Zebra Stone), Morganite with Azeztulite, Mount Shasta Opal, Rhodonite, Tangerose, Tanzine Aura Quartz, Tremolite, Tugtupite, Wind Fossil Agate, Xenotine. *Chakra:* solar plexus, heart

Bagua: see Feng Shui crystals page 295

Balance male/female energies: Alexandrite, Amphibole Quartz, Day and Night Quartz, Khutnohorite, Shiva Lingam. *Chakra:* base and sacral

Balance physical body with etheric: Ajoite, Andara Glass, Astraline, Eye of the Storm, Granite, Larvikite, Mohawkite, Nuummite, Rutile with Hematite, Sanda Rosa Azeztulite, Thompsonite. *Chakra:* dantien

Base chakra: Amber, Azurite, Bastnasite, Black Obsidian, Black Opal, Black Tourmaline, Bloodstone, Boji Stones, Candle Quartz, Carnelian, Chinese Red Quartz, Chrysocolla, Cinnabar Jasper, Citrine, Clinohumite, Cuprite, Dragon Stone, Eye of the Storm (Judy's Jasper), Fire Agate, Flint, Fulgarite, Gabbro, Garnet, Golden Topaz, Harlequin Quartz (Hematite in Quartz), Hematite, Kambaba Jasper, Keyiapo, Limonite, Obsidian, Pink Tourmaline, Poppy Jasper, Realgar and Orpiment, Red Amethyst, Red Calcite, Red Jasper, Red Zincite, Ruby, Serpentine, Serpentine in Obsidian, Shungite, Smoky Quartz, Sonora Sunrise, Spinel, Stromatolite, Tangerose, Triplite, Zircon. Place at perineum or base of spine.

> **balance and align:** Anandalite, Celestobarite, Green Ridge Quartz, Hematite Quartz, Red Calcite, Red Coral, Ruby, Shiva Lingam
>
> **spin too rapid/stuck open:** Agate, Green Ridge Quartz, Mahogany Obsidian, Pink Tourmaline, Smoky Quartz, Triplite in matrix
>
> **spin too sluggish/stuck closed:** Fire Agate, Hematite, Kundalini Quartz, Red Calcite, Serpentine, Sonora Sunrise, Triplite

Bathroom: Chlorite Quartz, Citrine, Okenite, Smoky Quartz

Beliefs that no longer serve, release: Ancestralite, Cradle of Humankind, Freedom Stone, Goethite, Lakelandite. *Chakra:* past life, third eye

Biological clock disturbances: Fluorapatite, Golden Healer Quartz, Kambaba Jasper, Menalite, Moonstone, Preseli Bluestone, Stromatolite. *Chakra:* dantien, higher heart, third eye or alta major (base of skull)

Biomagnetic field destabilized: Ajoite, Anandalite, Galena (wash hands after use, make essence by indirect method), Kyanite, Lepidolite, Magnetite, Orgonite, Preseli Bluestone, Quartz, Shungite, Sodalite, and see Aura page 261. *Chakra:* dantien, solar plexus

> **realign/strengthen:** Anandalite, Angelinite, Astraline, Celtic Quartz, Ethiopian Opal, Flint, Galena (wash hands after use, make essence by indirect method), Gold in Quartz, Golden Healer Quartz, Magnetite, Poldervaarite, Pollucite, Preseli Bluestone, Quantum

Quattro, Que Sera, Shungite, Sodalite

Blockages from past lives: Ajo Blue Calcite, Ancestralite, Flint, Freedom Stone, Lakelandite, Lemurian Seed, Nuummite, Orange Kyanite, Purple Scapolite, Rainbow Mayanite, Rhodozite, Serpentine in Obsidian. *Chakra:* past life, causal vortex

Blockages, self-imposed: Bowenite (New Jade), Brandenberg, Cradle of Humankind, Elestial Quartz, Freedom Stone, Gold Siberian Quartz, Prehnite with Epidote, Rhodozite, Serpentine in Obsidian, Sichuan Quartz. *Chakra:* higher heart

Blocked feelings: Frondellite, Indicolite Quartz, Lepidocrocite, Malachite, Mangano Calcite, Montebrasite, Obsidian, Peridot, Pyrite and Sphalerite, Pyrite in Quartz, Rainbow Mayanite, Rhodochrosite, Rhodonite, Tantalite, Tanzine Aura Quartz. *Chakra:* three-chambered heart, brow

Blueprint, etheric: Ammolite, Anandalite, Ancestralite, Andescine Labradorite, Astraline, Beryllonite, Black Kyanite, Brandenberg Amethyst, Chlorite Quartz, Cradle of Humankind, Ethiopian Opal, Eye of the Storm, Fulgarite, Golden Healer, Keyiapo, Khutnohorite, Lemurian Aquitane Calcite, Pollucite, Rhodozite, Ruby Lavender Quartz, Sanda Rosa Azeztulite, Scheelite, Seriphos Quartz, Tantalite. *Chakra:* soma, causal vortex

Body:

    acceptance of: Candle Quartz, Cradle of Humankind, Eye of the Storm, Phenacite, Vanadinite (wash hands after use, make essence by indirect method). *Chakra:*

earth, base, crown

discomfort at being in: Candle Quartz, Pearl Spa Dolomite, Quantum Quattro, Strontianite. *Chakra:* earth star, base, sacral, dantien

rebalance: Shiva Lingam, Shungite with Steatite, Victorite. *Chakra:* dantien

work efficiently: Golden Healer Quartz, Phlogopite

Boundaries: Brazilianite, Healer's Gold, Labradorite, Lemurian Jade, Serpentine in Obsidian, Tantalite. *Chakra:* solar plexus. (Or wear continuously.)

Break past life/ancestral patterns: Ancestralite, Arfvedsonite, Celadonite, Celtic Quartz, Cradle of Humankind, Freedom Stone, Garnet in Quartz, Green Ridge Quartz, Lemurian Seed, Owyhee Blue Opal, Porphyrite (Chinese Letter Stone), Rainbow Covellite, Rainbow Mayanite, Rhodozite, Scheelite, Shiva Shell, Stellar Beam Calcite

– C –

Cancer: Amethyst, Annabergite, Azeztulite, Azurite with Malachite, Bloodstone, Carnelian, Chalcopyrite, Champagne Aura Quartz, Cobaltite, Covellite, Cuprite with Chrysocolla, Diamond, Eilat Stone, Emerald, Fluorapatite, Fluorite, Gabbro, Gold in Quartz, Golden Healer Quartz, Green Ridge Quartz, Hematite, Heulandite, Kernite, Klinoptilolith, Lapis Lazuli, Lepidolite, Magnetite (Lodestone) with Smoky Quartz, Malachite, Malacolla, Melanite Garnet, Moonstone, Natrolite, Obsidian, Petalite, Pollucite, Quantum Quattro, Que Sera, Red Jasper, Reinerite, Rhodochrosite, Rhodozite, Sapphire, Scolecite, Selenite, Seraphinite, Shungite, Smoky Elestial Quartz, Smoky Quartz, Sodalite, Sonora Sunrise, Spinel, Stilbite, Sugilite, Thompsonite, Tourmaline, Ullmannite, Uvarovite, Xenotine. Place over site or appropriate chakra.

> **support during:** Amethyst Spirit Quartz, Bixbite, Black Diopside, Brandenberg Amethyst, Cassiterite, Cathedral Quartz, Cobalto Calcite, Dendritic Chalcedony, Epidote, Eye of the Storm, Green Ridge Quartz, Hemimorphite, Icicle Calcite, Lemurian Jade, Paraiba Tourmaline, Quantum Quattro, Que Sera, Reinerite, Rhodozite, Sonora Sunrise, Sugilite, Tremolite, Winchite

Car, neutralise EMFs: Black Tourmaline, Labradorite, Quartz, Shungite, Smoky Quartz. Keep in car.

Causal vortex chakra: Ammolite, Anandalite,

Ancestralite, Ajoite, Apatite, Azeztulite, Banded White Agate, Black or Blue Moonstone, Blue Kyanite, Brandenberg Amethyst, Chrysotile, Cobalto Calcite, Cradle of Humankind, Cryolite, Crystalline Blue Kyanite, Diamond, Diaspore (Zultanite), Fluorapatite, Freedom Stone, Herderite, Petalite, Phenacite, Preseli Bluestone, Rainbow Moonstone, Scolecite, Sugilite, Tanzanite. Place at base of skull.

   balance and align: Anandalite, Brandenberg Amethyst, Chrysotile, Crystalline Blue Kyanite, Fluorapatite, Phenacite, Preseli Bluestone, Scolecite, Smoky Elestial Quartz

   spin too rapid/stuck open: Black Moonstone, Cobalto Calcite, Diaspore, Scolecite with Natrolite

   spin too sluggish/stuck closed: Ajoite, Blue Moonstone, Herderite, Petalite, Tanzanite

Cell phones: Amazonite, Black Tourmaline, Diamond, Orgonite, Shieldite, Shungite, Smoky Elestial Quartz, Smoky Quartz, Sodalite. Tape to phone.

Cellular blueprint: Ajo Quartz, Ajoite, Ancestralite, Brandenberg Amethyst, Chlorite Quartz, Cradle of Humankind, Eye of the Storm, Fulgarite, Golden Healer, Kambaba Jasper, Keyiapo, Khutnohorite, Lakelandite, Rainbow Mayanite, Rhodozite, Ruby Lavender Quartz, Scheelite, Seriphos Quartz, Shattuckite, Shungite, Stromatolite, Yellow Kunzite. *Chakra:* higher heart, soma, alta major (base of skull) and see Karmic and Etheric body pages 309 and 293

Cellular memory: Ajo Quartz, Ajoite, Ancestralite,

Andean Blue Opal, Azotic Topaz, Brandenberg Amethyst, Bustamite, Chrysotile, Cradle of Humankind, Datolite, Dumortierite, Eilat Stone, Elestial Quartz, Eye of the Storm, Golden Healer, Heulandite, Leopardskin Jasper, Lepidocrocite, Nuummite, Rainbow Mayanite, Rhodozite, Sichuan Quartz, Smoky Quartz with Aegerine, Sodalite, Spirit Quartz, Valentinite and Stibnite. *Chakra:* dantien, alta major, causal vortex

Centring: Bloodstone, Calcite, Celestobarite, Coral, Eye of the Storm, Flint, Fossilised Wood, Garnet, Hematite, Kunzite, Obsidian, Onyx, Peanut Wood, Quartz, Red Jasper, Ruby, Sardonyx, Tourmalinated Quartz. *Chakra:* dantien

Chakra balance: Anandalite, Auralite 23, Black Kyanite, Citrine, Golden Healer Quartz, Lemurian Seed, Selenite, Sichuan Quartz

Chakra blockages: Ajo Quartz, Amechlorite, Anandalite, Black Kyanite, Chlorite Quartz, Cradle of Humankind, Eye of the Storm, Flint, Fulgarite, Golden Healer Quartz, Larvikite, Lemurian Seed, Picrolite, Prehnite with Epidote, Pyrite and Sphalerite, Rhodozite, Sanda Rosa Azeztulite, Seraphinite, Smoky Quartz with Aegerine, Shungite

Chakra cleanse: Anandalite, Enstatite and Diopside, Flint, Golden Healer Quartz, Graphic Smoky Quartz (Zebra Stone), Orange Kyanite, Novaculite, Nuummite, Rainbow Mayanite, Rhodozaz, Rhodozite, Shungite

Chakra detox: Anandalite, Chlorite Quartz, Eye of the Storm, Flint, Fulgarite, Golden Healer, Larvikite,

Seraphinite, Shungite, Smoky Quartz with Aegerine

Chakra energy leakage, prevent: Eudialyte, Gaspeite, Green Aventurine, Labradorite, Polychrome Jasper, Pyrite in Quartz, Tantalite, Thunder Egg. *Chakra:* dantien, spleen, solar plexus

Chakra entities, release: Anandalite, Eilat Stone, Flint, Holly Agate, Keyiapo, Klinoptilolith, Larvikite, Lemurian Seed, Novaculite, Pyromorphite, Rainbow Mayanite, Stibnite, and see Entity release page 292

Chakra mental influences, detach: Flint, Novaculite, Nuummite, Rainbow Mayanite

Chakra negative karma, disturbances from: Elestial Quartz, Golden Healer, Violane, Wind Fossil Agate. *Chakra:* earth, past life, alta major, causal vortex

Chakras, align with physical body: Anandalite, Celestial Quartz, Golden Healer, Keyiapo, Lemurian Jade, Lemurian Seed, Morion, Prasiolite, Preseli Bluestone, Rhodozite, Sichuan Quartz, Sillimanite, Smoky Herkimer Diamond, Thompsonite

Change, assimilate vibrational: Anandalite™, Bismuth, Candle Quartz, Ethiopian Opal, Lemurian Gold Opal, Sanda Rosa Azeztulite, Tangerose, Tugtupite with Nuummite. *Chakra:* Gaia gateway, causal vortex, stellar gateway

Change, facilitate: Celtic Quartz, Cradle of Humankind, Ethiopian Opal, Eudialyte, Fluorapatite, Freedom Stone, Golden Danburite, Heulandite, Luxullianite, Merlinite, Phenacite in Red Feldspar, Quantum Quattro, Scapolite, Shaman Quartz, Snakeskin Pyrite, Tangerine Dream

Lemurian. *Chakra:* heart, earth star

Change, ground: Aztee, Basalt, Boji Stones, Celtic Quartz, Champagne Aura Quartz, Empowerite, Kambaba Jasper, Lemurian Jade, Libyan Gold Tektite, Mohawkite, Nunderite, Peanut Wood, Petrified Wood, Polychrome Jasper, Preseli Bluestone, Schalenblende, Serpentine in Obsidian, Smoky Amethyst, Smoky Herkimer, Smoky Quartz, Stromatolite, Tibetan Black Spot Quartz. *Chakra:* earth star, dantien

Change, psychological: Annabergite, Elestial Quartz, Frondellite, Lilac Crackle Quartz. *Chakra:* causal vortex

Channelling, protection during: Angelite, Labradorite, Petalite, Tantalite

Chemical pollution: Amber, Chlorite Quartz, Granite, Halite, Hanksite, Pumice, Quantum Quattro, Shungite, Smoky Elestial Quartz, Smoky Quartz, Tantalite

Chemotherapy support: Agrellite, Eye of the Storm, Klinoptilolith, Shungite, Tremolite, Winchite

Childbirth, protect during: Ammolite, Ammonite, Chrysocolla, Eye of the Storm, Geodes, Hematite, Lepidolite, Malachite, Menalite, Moonstone, Picture Jasper, Rose Quartz

Children, protect: Amber, Amethyst, Black Tourmaline, Bloodstone, Blue Lace Agate, Carnelian, Eye of the Storm (Judy's Jasper), Green Moss Agate, Jade, Peach Aventurine, Polychrome Jasper, Rhodolite Garnet, Ruby, Selenite, Shungite, Turquoise

Chronic:

   conditions: Apricot Quartz, Bismuth, Diopside

disease: Apricot Quartz, Bismuth, Cathedral Quartz, Lemurian Jade, Orgonite, Petrified Wood, Quantum Quattro, Que Sera, Shungite, Witches Finger. *Chakra:* dantien

exhaustion: Apricot Quartz, Bismuth, Bronzite, Cinnabar in Jasper, Eye of the Storm, Poppy Jasper, Prehnite with Epidote, Triplite, Trummer Jasper. *Chakra:* dantien, higher heart

fatigue syndrome: Adamite, Amethyst, Ametrine, Apricot Quartz, Aquamarine, Aragonite, Barite, Chrysotile in Serpentine, Citrine, Green Tourmaline, Orange Calcite, Petrified Wood, Pyrite in Quartz, Quartz, Rhodochrosite, Ruby, Shungite, Tourmaline, Triplite, Trummer Jasper, Zincite. *Chakra:* dantien, and see ME, page 313

illness: Cat's Eye, Danburite, Dendritic Chalcedony, Golden Danburite, Petrified Wood, Poppy Jasper, Que Sera, Shungite, Trummer Jasper. *Chakra:* earth star, solar plexus, higher heart

Clearing 'bad vibes': Amazonite, Amber, Amethyst, Aventurine, Black Tourmaline, Chlorite Quartz, Fluorite, Fulgarite, Graphic Smoky Quartz, Iron Pyrite, Kyanite, Lepidolite, Magnetite, Quartz, Rose Quartz, Selenite, Shieldite, Shungite, Smoky Elestial Quartz, Smoky Quartz, Tantalite, Tektite

Close down and ground: Agate, Black Tourmaline, Bloodstone, Boji Stones, Dravite (Brown) Tourmaline, Fire Agate, Galena (wash hands after use, make essence by indirect method), Hematite, Magnetite, Obsidian,

Smoky Quartz, Sodalite, Tourmalinated Quartz, Unakite. *Chakra:* base or earth star

Codependency: Bytownite, Dumortierite, Fenster Quartz, Quantum Quattro, Sichuan Quartz, Vera Cruz Amethyst, Xenotine. *Chakra:* base, dantien, causal vortex

Computer stress: Amazonite, Amber, Aventurine, Chlorite Quartz, Eye of the Storm, Fluorite, Fulgarite, Galena (wash hands after use, make essence by indirect method), Lepidolite, Orgonite, Purple Sugilite, Rose Quartz, Shieldite, Shungite, Smoky Quartz, Sodalite, Sugilite, Tektite. *Chakra:* higher heart

Confidence: Candle Quartz, Dumortierite, Erythrite, Eudialyte, Jasper, Kakortokite, Lazulite, Morion, Prasiolite, Purpurite, Strontianite. *Chakra:* base, dantien

Conflict resolution: Champagne Aura Quartz, Fluorapatite, Rose Quartz, Trigonic Quartz. *Chakra:* causal vortex

Confusion, disperse: Blue Scapolite, Celestial Quartz, Crystal Cap Amethyst, Elestial Quartz, Gabbro, Hematoid Calcite, Lepidocrocite, Limonite, Kakortokite, Owyhee Blue Opal, Paraiba Tourmaline. *Chakra:* between third eye and soma

Contracts, renegotiate: Anandalite, Ancestralite, Boli Stone, Cradle of Humankind, Dumortierite, Freedom Stone, Gabbro, Nuummite, Prasiolite, Purple Scapolite, Quantum Quattro, Red Amethyst, Shiva Lingam. *Chakra:* past life, alta major, causal vortex

Contraindications and cautions:

   Bronzite: Use with caution as it rebounds negative

energy back and forth, amplifying it. Combine with Black Tourmaline or Smoky Quartz.

catharsis, may induce: Barite, Epidote, Hypersthene, Smoky Spirit Quartz, Tugtupite (replace with Quantum Quattro or Smoky Quartz)

epilepsy: Dumortierite, Goethite, Zircon

giddiness, remove if causes: Banded Agate

heart palpitations, if causes remove: Eilat Stone, Malachite

illusion, may induce: Blue or Rainbow Moonstone

negative energy heightened if worn constantly: Epidote, Hypersthene

potentially toxic: The following crystals may contain traces of potentially toxic minerals although these are bound up within the structure (use polished stone, make crystal essence by indirect method, wash hands after handling):

Actinolite, Adamite, Ajoite, Alexandrite, Almandine Garnet, Amazonite, Andaluscite, Aquamarine, Aragonite, Arsenopyrite, Atacamite, Aurichalcite, Axinite, Azurite, Beryl, Beryllium, Biotite (ferrous), Bixbite, Black Tourmaline, Boji Stones, Bornite, Brazilianite, Brochantite, Bumble Bee Jasper, Cassiterite, Cavansite, Celestite, Celtic Quartz, Cerussite, Cervanite, Chalchantite, Chalcopyrite (Peacock Ore), Chrysoberyl, Chrysocolla, Chrysotile, Cinnabar, Conichalcite, Copper, Covellite, Crocoite, Cryolite, Cuprite, Diopside, Dioptase, Dumortierite, Emerald, Epidote, Galena, Garnet, Garnierite

(Falcondoite), Gem Silica, Germanium, Goshenite, Heliodor, Hessonite Garnet, Hiddenite, Iolite, Jadeite, Jamesonite, Kinoite, Klinoptilolith, Kunzite, Kyanite, Labradorite, Lapis Lazuli, Lazurite, Lepidolite, Magnetite, Malachite, Malacolla, Marcasite, Messina Quartz, Mohawkite, Moldavite, Moonstone, Moqui Balls, Morganite, Orpiment, Pargasite, Piemontite, Pietersite, Plancheite, Prehnite, Psilomelane, Pyrite, Pyromorphite, Quantum Quattro, Que Sera, Realgar, Realgar and Orpiment, Renierite, Rhodolite Garnet, Ruby, Sapphire, Serpentine, Smithsonite, Sodalite, Spessartine Garnet, Sphalerite, Spinel, Spodumene, Staurolite, Stibnite, Stilbite, Sugilite, Sulphur, Sunstone, Tanzanite, Tiffany Stone, Tiger's Eye, Topaz, Torbernite, Tourmaline, Tremolite, Turquoise, Uranophane, Uvarovite Garnet, Valentinite, Vanadinite, Variscite, Vesuvianite, Vivianite, Wavellite, Wulfenite, Zircon, Zoisite

psychiatric conditions, paranoia or schizophrenia: 277 Do not use crystals unless under the supervision of a qualified crystal healer.

radioactive: Very dark Smoky Quartz, Uranophane (use under supervision)

toehold in incarnation: Avoid Gabbro with Moonstone, Llanite (Llanoite), Polychrome Jasper. *Chakra:* earth star and soma

Cord cutting: Banded Agate, Charoite (raw), Dumortierite, Flint, Green Aventurine, Green Obsidian, Jasper Knife, Laser Quartz, Leopardskin Jasper,

Malachite, Novaculite, Petalite, Pietersite, Rainbow Aura Quartz, Rainbow Mayanite, Rainbow Obsidian, Smoky Brandenberg Amethyst, Stibnite, Sunstone, Wulfenite. *Chakra:* past life, causal vortex, spleen, solar plexus, third eye, base and sacral. 'Comb' all over aura.

Cravings: see Addictions page 256

Crime, protection against: Jet, Sardonyx

Crown chakra: Afghanite, Amethyst, Amphibole Quartz, Anandalite, Angelite, Angel's Wing Calcite, Arfvedsonite, Auralite 23, Brandenberg Amethyst, Celestial Quartz, Celtic Quartz, Citrine, Clear Tourmaline, Golden Beryl, Golden Healer, Green Ridge Quartz, Larimar, Lepidolite, Moldavite, Novaculite, Petalite, Phenacite, Purple Jasper, Purple Sapphire, Quartz, Rosophia, Satyamani and Satyaloka Quartz, Selenite, Serpentine, Titanite (Sphene), Trigonic, White Calcite, White Topaz. *Chakra:* crown

> **balance and align:** Amethyst, Anandalite, Auralite 23, Brandenberg Amethyst, Phenacite, Selenite, Sugilite
>
> **spin too rapid/stuck open:** Amethyst, Amphibole Quartz, Larimar, Petalite, Serpentine, White Calcite
>
> **spin too sluggish/stuck closed:** Anandalite, Moldavite, Phenacite, Rosophia, Selenite

Crystals that rarely require cleansing: Citrine, Kyanite. (Note: cleansing is recommended for all crystals, see pages 11, 21.)

Crystals that require daily cleansing: Shungite

Curses, break ancestral: Black Tourmaline, Nuummite, Purpurite, Quantum Quattro, Shattuckite, Stibnite, Tiger's Eye, Tourmalinated Quartz. *Chakra:* past life, throat, third eye, causal vortex

Curses, deflect effects of: Black Tourmaline, Bronzite (use with caution may rebound), Green Ridge Quartz, Quantum Quattro, Shungite, Tourmalinated Quartz. *Chakra:* past life, throat, causal vortex

Curses, remove: Black Tourmaline, Flint, Nuummite, Purpurite, Quantum Quattro, Rainbow Mayanite, Shattuckite, Shungite, Stibnite, Tiger's Eye, Tourmalinated Quartz. *Chakra:* heart, solar plexus, third eye, causal vortex

Curses, turn back: Black Tourmaline, Bronzite (use with caution), Master Shamanite, Mohawkite, Nuummite, Richterite, Tantalite, Tourmalinated Quartz. *Chakra:* throat

– D –

Dantien: Amber, Carnelian, Chinese Red Quartz, Condor Agate, Empowerite, Eye of the Storm, Fire Agate, Fire Opal, Golden Herkimer, Green Ridge Quartz, Hematite, Hematoid Calcite, Kambaba Jasper, Madagascan Red Celestial Quartz, Moonstone, Orange River Quartz, Peanut Wood, Polychrome Jasper, Poppy Jasper, Red Amethyst, Red Jasper, Rhodozite, Rose or Ruby Aura Quartz, Rosophia, Stromatolite, Topaz, Triplite

> **balance and align:** Empowerite, Eye of the Storm, Green Ridge Quartz, Poppy Jasper
>
> **spin too rapid/stuck open:** Peanut Wood, Polychrome Jasper, Stromatolite
>
> **spin too sluggish/stuck closed:** Fire Agate, Fire Opal, Hematite, Madagascan Red Celestial Quartz, Poppy Jasper, Red Jasper, Triplite

De-cursing kit: Novaculite and Nuummite, Tourmalinated Quartz, and see Uncursing page 348

Defensive walls, dismantle: Calcite Fairy Stone, Cradle of Humankind, Rhodochrosite (to replace with interface see page 308)

'Demonic possession': Dravite (Brown) Tourmaline, Jet, Smoky Amethyst

Depression, anti: Ajo Blue Calcite, Amber, Amethyst, Ametrine, Apatite, Apophyllite Botswana Agate, Carnelian, Chrysoprase, Citrine, Clinohumite, Dianite, Eisenkiesel, Eudialyte, Flint, Garnet, Golden Healer, Green Ridge Quartz, Hematite, Idocrase, Jade, Jet,

Kunzite, Lapis Lazuli, Lepidolite, Lithium Quartz, Macedonian Opal, Maw Sit Sit, Montebrasite, Moss Agate, Orange Kyanite, Pink Sunstone, Porphyrite (Chinese Letter Stone), Purple Tourmaline, Rainbow Goethite, Rutilated Quartz, Siberian Quartz, Sillimanite, Smoky Quartz, Spessartine Garnet, Spider Web Obsidian, Spinel, Staurolite, Sunstone, Tiger's Eye, Tugtupite, Turquoise, Witches Finger. *Chakra:* solar plexus. Wear continuously.

Detoxification: Amber, Amechlorite, Amethyst, Anhydrite, Apache Tear, Aventurine, Azurite, Banded Agate, Barite, Bastnasite, Bloodstone, Chalk, Chlorite, Chlorite Quartz, Chrysoprase, Conichalcite, Coprolite, Covellite, Cuprite with Chrysocolla, Dendritic Agate, Diaspore, Emerald, Eye of the Storm, Fire Obsidian, Galena (wash hands after use, make essence by indirect method), Golden Danburite, Golden Healer Quartz, Graphic Smoky Quartz, Green Garnet, Greensand, Halite, Hanksite, Herkimer Diamond, Hypersthene, Iolite, Jade, Jamesonite, Jet, Kambaba Jasper, Larvikite, Malachite, Merlinite, Mica, Obsidian, Ocean Jasper, Orgonite, Phlogopite, Poppy Jasper, Pumice, Quantum Quattro, Que Sera, Rainbow Covellite, Richterite, Ruby, Seraphinite, Shungite, Smoky Elestial Quartz, Smoky Quartz, Smoky Quartz with Aegerine, Stilbite, Sulphur, Sulphur in Quartz, Thunder Egg, Tiger's Eye, Topaz, Tree Agate, Turquoise, Zoisite. *Chakra:* solar plexus, earth star, base. Or place in environment.

Detoxify body: Amechlorite, Banded Agate, Barite,

Conichalcite, Coprolite, Diaspore (Zultanite), Eye of the Storm, Golden Danburite, Golden Healer, Halite, Hanksite, Hematite, Hypersthene, Jamesonite, Larvikite, Pumice, Rainbow Covellite, Richterite, Shungite, Smoky Herkimer, Smoky Quartz, Smoky Quartz with Aegerine. *Chakra:* solar plexus, earth star, base

Detoxify emotions: Golden Danburite, Golden Healer, Morganite with Azeztulite, Rhodonite, Spirit Quartz. *Chakra:* solar plexus

Detoxify etheric body: Anandalite, Astraline, Brandenberg Amethyst, Ethiopian Opal, Eye of the Storm, Frondellite with Strengite, Golden Healer, Lemurian Aquitane Calcite, Seriphos Quartz, Shungite, Spirit Quartz, Tantalite. *Chakra:* third eye

Detoxify mind: Auralite 23, Fluorite, Golden Healer, Thunder Egg. *Chakra:* third eye

Detoxify spiritual body: Anandalite, Eye of the Storm, Golden Danburite, Spirit Quartz. *Chakra:* crown

Dining room: Citrine, Jasper

Disconnection from earth: Basalt, Flint, Granite, Hematite, Kambaba Jasper, Lemurian Jade, Libyan Gold Tektite, Moldavite, Preseli Bluestone, Smoky Elestial Quartz, Stromatolite, Strontianite. *Chakra:* earth star, Gaia gateway, dantien, soma

Disease/illness, protect against: Bloodstone, Carnelian, Cavansite, Chalcopyrite, Jade, Jet, Quantum Quattro, Que Sera, Zircon

Disembodied spirits attached to places: Larimar, Marcasite, Quartz, Smoky Amethyst (effect is enhanced if you add Petaltone Astral Clear which directs the spirit to the light)

Dysfunctional patterns, dissolve: Alunite, Arfvedsonite, Celadonite, Dumortierite, Fenster Quartz, Freedom Stone, Garnet in Quartz, Glendonite, Golden Healer, Rainbow Covellite, Scheelite, Spider Web Obsidian, Stellar Beam Calcite

Earth, attune to: Chrysocolla, Granite, Hematite, Hiddenite, Preseli Bluestone

Earth healing: Ammolite, Aragonite, Atlantasite, Black Diopside, Black Tourmaline, Blue Sapphire, Brown Aragonite, Bustamite, Cacoxenite, Celestial Quartz, Champagne Aura Quartz, Chlorite Quartz, Desert Rose, Dragon Stone, Eye of the Storm, Feldspar, Flint, Fulgarite, Granite, Golden or Tangerine Lemurians, Green Ridge Quartz, Greenlandite, Kambaba Jasper, Labradorite, Lemurian Jade, Marble, Mohawkite, Monazite, Prehnite, Preseli Bluestone, Quartz, Rhodozite, Scolecite, Selenite, Seriphos Quartz, Smoky Brandenberg, Smoky Elestial, Smoky Quartz, Specular Hematite, Stromatolite, Super 7, Tantalite, Thunder Egg, Torbernite, Witches Finger, Z-stone. *Chakra:* earth star. Place in environment.

Earth star chakra: Agnitite™, Atlantasite, Basalt, Boji Stones, Brown Jasper, Celestobarite, Champagne Aura Quartz, Cuprite, Fire Agate, Flint, Galena (wash hands after use, make essence by indirect method), Golden Herkimer, Granite, Graphic Smoky Quartz, Hematite, Lemurian Jade, Limonite, Madagascan Red Celestial Quartz, Mahogany Obsidian, Proustite, Red Amethyst, Rhodonite, Rhodozite, Rosophia, Smoky Elestial Quartz, Smoky Quartz, Thunder Egg, Tourmaline. Place below feet.

    balance and align: Blue Flint, Brown-flash

Anandalite, Green Ridge Quartz, Hematite, Smoky Elestial Quartz

spin too rapid/stuck open: Flint, Graphic Smoky Quartz, Green Ridge Quartz, Smoky Quartz

spin too sluggish/stuck closed: Golden Herkimer, Hematite, Red Amethyst, Rhodozite, Thunder Egg

Electrical systems of body, rebalance: Amber, Amblygonite, Cavansite, Galena (wash hands after use, make essence by indirect method), Golden Healer Quartz, Lepidolite, Montebrasite, Orgonite, Pollucite, Quartz, Shiva Lingam, Shungite, Sodalite, Tourmaline

Electrolytes, nerve and muscle function: Coral, Malachite, Native Copper, Quartz

Electromagnetic:

antidote: Ajoite in Shattuckite, Amazonite, Amber, Auralite 23, Aventurine, Black Moonstone, Black Tourmaline, Black Tourmaline in Quartz, Blizzard Stone, Bloodstone, Chlorite Quartz, Diamond, Flint, Fluorapatite, Fluorite, Fulgarite, Gabbro, Galena (wash hands after use, make essence by indirect method), Graphic Smoky Quartz, Herkimer Diamond, Jasper, Klinoptilolith, Lepidolite, Malachite, Native Copper, Natrolite, Obsidian, Orgonite, Phlogopite, Pollucite, Pyrite in Quartz, Quartz, Quantum Quattro, Que Sera, Red Amethyst, Rose Quartz, Scolecite, Shieldite, Shungite, Smoky Quartz, Sodalite, Stilbite, Thompsonite, Thunder Egg, Yellow Kunzite

field, computer: Amazonite, Amethyst, Black Tourmaline, Fluorite, Green or Brown Jasper,

Herkimer Diamond, Jet, Lepidolite, large Diamonds, Malachite, Obsidian, Shungite, Smoky Quartz, Sodalite, Turquoise, Yellow Kunzite. Place on or near the computer or wear over higher heart chakra.

field, regulate personal: Ajoite in Shattuckite, Amazonite, Amber, Auralite 23, Black Moonstone, Champagne Aura Quartz, Eye of the Storm, Fluorapatite, Fluorite, Fulgarite, Gabbro, Galena (wash hands after use, make essence by indirect method), Golden Healer Quartz, Montebrasite, Poppy Jasper, Preseli Bluestone, Quantum Quattro, Que Sera, Rose Quartz, Shungite, Tourmaline, Turquoise. *Chakra:* earth star, base. Or place in environment.

pollution, protect against: Ajoite in Shattuckite, Amazonite, Amber, Andara Glass, Black Moonstone, Black Tourmaline, Blizzard Stone, Champagne Aura Quartz, Chlorite Quartz, Diamond, Flint, Fluorite, Gabbro, Galena (wash hands after use, make essence by indirect method), Graphic Smoky Quartz, Hackmanite, Herkimer Diamond, Klinoptilolith, Kunzite, Lepidolite, Malachite, Marble, Morion, Native Copper, Orgonite, Phlogopite, Poppy Jasper, Quartz, Que Sera, Red Amethyst, Rose Quartz, Shieldite, Shungite, Smoky Elestial Quartz, Smoky Herkimer Diamond, Smoky Quartz, Sodalite, Tantalite, Thunder Egg. *Chakra:* earth star, base. Or place in environment or around house.

Electrostatic: Amber, Halite, Hanksite, Jet, Quartz, Tourmaline

Emotional abuse: Azeztulite with Morganite, Cobalto Calcite, Eilat Stone, Golden Healer, Lazurine, Pink Crackle Quartz, Proustite, Tugtupite. *Chakra:* sacral, heart

Emotional attachments: Aegerine, Ajoite, Drusy Golden Healer, Ilmenite, Novaculite, Nuummite, Pink Lemurian Seed, Rainbow Mayanite, Smoky Amethyst, Stibnite, Tantalite, Tinguaite. *Chakra:* past life, causal vortex, base or sacral

Emotional baggage: Ajoite, Frondellite plus Strengite, Golden Healer Quartz, Rose Elestial Quartz, Tangerose. *Chakra:* solar plexus

Emotional balance: Amblygonite, Dalmation Stone, Eilat Stone

Emotional black hole: Ajoite, Cobalto Calcite, Quantum Quattro. *Chakra:* higher heart

Emotional blackmail: Tugtupite and see Cord cutting page 277. *Chakra:* solar plexus

Emotional blockages from past lives: Aegerine, Datolite, Dumortierite, Frondellite plus Strengite, Graphic Smoky Quartz (Zebra Stone), Prehnite with Epidote, Pyrite and Sphalerite, Quantum Quattro, Rainbow Obsidian, Rhodozite, Rose Elestial Quartz, Serpentine in Obsidian. *Chakra:* past life, three-chambered heart, causal vortex, and see Past life/ancestral healing page 319

Emotional body: Cobalto Calcite, Golden Healer, Mangano Calcite, Oregon Opal, Rhodochrosite

Emotional bondage: Ajoite, Cradle of Humankind, Freedom Stone, Frondellite plus Strengite. *Chakra:* solar plexus

Emotional bonds in relationships, disconnect: Amblygonite, Brandenberg Amethyst, Cradle of Humankind, Flint, Green Aventurine, Rainbow Mayanite, Shiva Lingam, Stibnite, Tugtupite, Wind Fossil Agate. *Chakra:* spleen, solar plexus, base and sacral, and see Cord cutting page 277

Emotional conditioning, release: Clevelandite, Drusy Golden Healer, Golden Healer Quartz. *Chakra:* solar plexus, third eye

Emotional debris: Ajoite, Hematite, Pink Lemurian Seed, Rainbow Mayanite, Shiva Shell, Smoky Elestial Quartz. *Chakra:* solar plexus

Emotional dependency: Cobalto Calcite and see Cord cutting page 277. *Chakra:* base

Emotional equilibrium: Adamite, Merlinite, Quantum Quattro, Rutile with Hematite, Shungite

Emotional hooks, remove: Amblygonite, Cradle of Humankind, Drusy Golden Healer, Freedom Stone, Goethite, Golden Danburite, Green Aventurine, Klinoptilolith, Novaculite, Nunderite, Nuummite, Orange Kyanite, Pyromorphite, Rainbow Mayanite, Tantalite, Tugtupite. *Chakra:* solar plexus, spleen

Emotional manipulation: Pink Lemurian Seed, Tantalite. *Chakra:* sacral, solar plexus, third eye, spleen

Emotional maturation: Alexandrite, Cobalto Calcite

Emotional pain: Blue Euclase, Cobalto Calcite, Golden Healer, Mangano Calcite, Morganite, Morganite with Azeztulite, Rhodochrosite, Rhodonite, Rose Quartz. *Chakra:* past life, heart, higher heart, solar plexus

Emotional pain after separation: Aegerine, Eilat Stone, Golden Healer, Mangano Calcite, Rhodonite, Rose Quartz, Tugtupite. *Chakra:* higher heart

Emotional patterns: Arfvedsonite, Brandenberg Amethyst, Celadonite, Fenster Quartz, Rainbow Covellite, Scheelite. *Chakra:* solar plexus, base

Emotional release: Cobalto Calcite, Golden Healer, Malachite. *Chakra:* solar plexus, base, sacral

Emotional shut down, release: Ice Quartz

Emotional stability/strength: Mohawkite. *Chakra:* base

Emotional toxicity: Ajoite, Arsenopyrite, Banded Agate, Champagne Aura Quartz, Drusy Danburite with Chlorite, Golden Healer, Valentinite and Stibnite

Emotional turmoil: Cobalto Calcite, Desert Rose, Eye of the Storm, Golden Healer, Mangano Calcite, Rose Quartz. *Chakra:* base

Emotional underlying causes of distress: Eye of the Storm, Gaia Stone, Lemurian Gold Opal, Richterite, Riebekite with Sugilite and Bustamite, Smoky Amethyst. *Chakra:* solar plexus, past life

Emotional wounds: Ajo Quartz, Eudialyte, Fiskenaesset Ruby, Golden Healer, Macedonian Opal, Mangano Calcite, Moldau Quartz, Mookaite Jasper, Prehnite with Epidote, Rathbunite™, Rose Quartz, Rosophia, Scheelite, Tangerose, Tugtupite, Xenotine. *Chakra:* past life, heart, higher heart, solar plexus

Emotional/ancestral trauma: Ajo Blue Calcite, Ajoite, Ancestralite, Blue Euclase, Cavansite, Cobalto Calcite, Cradle of Humankind, Empowerite, Epidote, Freedom

Stone, Gaia Stone, Golden Healer, Graphic Smoky Quartz, Guinea Fowl Jasper, Holly Agate, Mangano Vesuvianite, Oceanite, Orange River Quartz, Oregon Opal, Peanut Wood, Ruby Lavender Quartz, Sea Sediment Jasper, Tantalite, Tugtupite, Victorite. *Chakra:* solar plexus, past life

Ending a relationship positively: Blue Topaz, Pietersite, Rhodochrosite, Rose Quartz. *Chakra:* heart

Endocrine system: Adamite, Alexandrite, Amber, Amechlorite, Amethyst, Aquamarine, Azeztulite with Morganite, Black Moonstone, Bloodstone, Blue Quartz, Bustamite, Champagne Aura Quartz, Chrysoberyl, Citrine, Fire Agate, Fire and Ice Quartz, Golden Healer, Golden Topaz, Green Calcite, Green Obsidian, Howlite, Magnetite, Menalite, Pargasite, Pentagonite, Peridot, Picrolite, Pietersite, Pink Heulandite, Pink Tourmaline, Poppy Jasper, Quantum Quattro, Que Sera, Rhodochrosite, Richterite, Ruby Aura Quartz, Seriphos Quartz, Smoky Amethyst, Sodalite, Topaz, Tourmaline, Trummer Jasper, Yellow Jasper. *Chakra:* dantien, higher heart

Energetic well-being: Cinnabar Jasper, Fire Agate, Golden Healer Quartz, Jamesonite, Poppy Jasper, Quantum Quattro, Que Sera, Tantalite, Trummer Jasper

Energy: Agate, Amber, Apophyllite, Aragonite, Bloodstone, Blue Goldstone, Calcite, Carnelian, Coral, Danburite, Fire Agate, Green Jasper, Hematite, Jasper, Peridot, Prehnite, Quantum Quattro, Quartz, Que Sera, Rhodochrosite, Ruby, Rutilated Quartz, Strawberry

Lemurian, Triplite. *Chakra:* base, sacral, dantien. Or place in environment.

amplify: Poppy Jasper, Preseli Bluestone, Ruby Lavender Quartz, Sedona Stone, Triplite. *Chakra:* base, dantien

blockages: Charoite, Danburite, Flint, Fulgarite, Labradorite, Lemurian Quartz

depletion, reverse: Eudialyte, Fire Opal, Healer's Gold, Labradorite, Macedonian Opal, Pink Sunstone, Poppy Jasper, Preseli Bluestone, Que Sera, Red Jasper, Ruby Lavender Quartz, Rutilated Quartz, Scheelite, Sedona Stone, Strawberry Lemurian. *Chakra:* dantien

energetic cleanse: Amber, Anandalite, Merlinite

field, strengthen: Garnet, Healer's Gold, Kunzite, Labradorite, Mohawkite, Poppy Jasper, Preseli Bluestone, Quartz, Ruby Lavender Quartz. Chakra: dantien, solar plexus

imbalances: Lepidocrocite

leakage from aura: Amber, Flint, Healer's Gold, Labradorite, Molybdenite in Quartz, Nuummite, Pyrite in Quartz, Rainbow Mayanite, Strawberry Lemurian, Tantalite. *Chakra:* dantien, higher heart

stagnant: Black Tourmaline, Calcite, Clear Topaz, Graphic Smoky Quartz, Smoky Elestial Quartz, Smoky Quartz

system: Garnet in Quartz. *Chakra:* dantien

unbalanced field: Amber, Garnet in Quartz, Goldsheen Obsidian, Preseli Bluestone, Ruby in Zoisite

Entities attached to places: Celtic Quartz, Jasper Knife, Larimar, Lemurian Seed, Marcasite, Quartz *with Petaltone Astral Clear*, Smoky Amethyst

Entities attached to third eye: Anandalite, Brandenberg Amethyst, Celestobarite, Flint, Larimar, Laser Quartz, Lemurian Seed, Petalite, Pyroluscite, Shattuckite, Smoky Amethyst, Smoky Phantom

Entities, release from chakras: Flint, Lemurian Seed, Petalite, Smoky Amethyst

Entities, remove attached: Anandalite, Drusy Golden Healer, Flint, Klinoptilolith, Larvikite, Lemurian Seed, Nirvana Quartz, Phantom Selenite, Pyromorphite, Rainbow Mayanite, Smoky Amethyst, Stibnite. *Chakra:* sacral, solar plexus, third eye

Environment, improve: Amazonite, Aragonite, Black Tourmaline, Chlorite Quartz, Eye of the Storm, Golden Healer Quartz, Malachite, Orgonite, Poppy Jasper, Quartz, Rose Quartz, Selenite, Smoky Quartz, White or Rose Elestial Quartz and see Earth healing page 284

Environmental:

> **diseases:** Chlorite Quartz, Drusy Quartz on Sphalerite, Eye of the Storm, Feldspar, Golden Healer Quartz, Marble, Orgonite, Petrified Wood, Poppy Jasper, Preseli Bluestone, Quartz, Shieldite, Shungite, Smoky Elestial Quartz, and see Geopathic Stress page 299. *Chakra:* earth star. Or place in environment.

> **harmony:** Khutnohorite, Rose Quartz, Sardonyx, Selenite

> **pollution:** Alunite, Amber, Anhydrite, Black

Tourmaline, Champagne Aura Quartz, Chlorite Quartz, Eye of the Storm, Flint, Golden Healer Quartz, Graphic Smoky Quartz, Halite, Hanksite, Labradorite, Moss Agate, Orgonite, Phlogopite, Poppy Jasper, Que Sera, Selenite, Shieldite, Shungite, Smoky Elestial Quartz, Smoky Quartz, Sulphur, Sulphur in Quartz, Tantalite, Thunder Egg, Trummer Jasper, Zincite. *Chakra:* earth star. Place stones in earth or around house.

Envy, ameliorate: Blood of Isis, Carnelian. *Chakra:* solar plexus, heart

Etheric blueprint: Ajoite, Anandalite, Andescine Labradorite, Angelinite, Apatite, Astraline, Black Spot Quartz, Brandenberg Amethyst, Cathedral Quartz, Chrysocolla, Chrysotile, Cradle of Humankind, Elestial Quartz, Ethiopian Opal, Eye of the Storm, Flint, Girasol, Golden Healer, Herkimer Diamond, Keyiapo, Khutnohorite, Kunzite, Laser Quartz, Lemurian Aquitane Calcite, Merlinite, Novaculite, Phantom Quartz, Phenacite, Rhodozite, Ruby Lavender Quartz, Sanda Rosa Azeztulite, Scheelite, Selenite, Sichuan Quartz, Smoky Elestial, Spirit Quartz, Stellar Beam Calcite, Tangerine Dream Lemurian, Tangerine Quartz, Tantalite, Tanzine Aura Quartz, Tibetan Quartz. *Chakra:* causal vortex, past life

Etheric body, realign/strengthen: Anandalite, Angelinite, Astraline, Ethiopian Opal, Gold in Quartz, Golden Healer Quartz, Golden Selenite, Green Ridge Quartz

Etheric pests: Cryolite, Tantalite and see Aura page 262

Etheric support: Eye of the Storm, Mohawkite, Tantalite, Tremolite, Winchite

Ethnic conflict: Afghanite, Azeztulite with Morganite, Catlinite, Champagne Aura Quartz, Chinese Red Quartz, Fluorapatite, Trigonic Quartz, Tugtupite

Everyday reality, difficulty in dealing with: Blue Halite, Bornite, Cathedral Quartz, Dumortierite, Lepidocrocite, Marcasite, Neptunite, Pearl Spa Dolomite, Purpurite. *Chakra:* earth star, dantien. Or wear continuously.

Evil eye, protect against: Agate, Banded Agate, Black Tourmaline, Carnelian, Cat's Eye, Eye Agate, Jet, Malachite, Topaz

Evil, protect against: Agate, Beryl, Black Tourmaline, Blue Chalcedony, Eye Agate, Eye of the Storm, Garnet, Halite, Hanksite, Herkimer Diamond, Jet, Malachite, Pyrite, Quartz, Sapphire, Snowflake Obsidian, Tiger Iron, Turquoise

Exhaustion: Bismuth, Carnelian, Chlorite Quartz, Cinnabar Jasper, Cuprite with Chrysocolla, Epidote, Eye of the Storm, Fire Opal, Garnet, Golden Healer Quartz, Hematite, Lepidolite, Pietersite, Poppy Jasper, Quantum Quattro, Red Jasper, Ruby, Rutilated Quartz, Scheelite, Sulphur, Tiger Iron, Triplite, Turquoise. *Chakra:* base

– F –

Family burdens: Golden Healer, Mohawkite, Polychrome Jasper, Tinguaite

Family scapegoat: Blue Lace Agate, Celtic Chevron Quartz, Celtic Golden Healer, Green Tourmaline, Larimar, Ocean Jasper, Rose Quartz Scapolite, Tree Agate. *Chakra:* causal vortex, base

Family stress: Candle Quartz, Chinese Red Quartz, Datolite, Eye of the Storm, Faden Quartz, Fairy Quartz, Glendonite, Golden Healer, Mohave Turquoise, Riebekite with Sugilite and Bustamite, Shaman Quartz, Shungite, Spirit Quartz. *Chakra:* solar plexus, base and sacral

Family ties, strengthen: Cat's Eye Quartz, Glendonite, Polychrome Jasper. *Chakra:* solar plexus

Fear, irrational from past lives: Freedom Stone, Revelation Stone

Fear, of the unknown: Bastnasite

Fear, overcome: Amazonite, Aquamarine, Arsenopyrite, Blue Quartz, Cacoxenite, Carolite, Dumortierite, Eilat Stone, Graphic Smoky Quartz (Zebra Stone), Guardian Stone, Hackmanite, Icicle Calcite, Khutnohorite, Leopardskin Jasper, Moss Agate, Oceanite, Paraiba Tourmaline, Red and Orange Calcite, Rose Quartz, Spectrolite, Spirit Quartz, Tangerose, Thunder Egg, Tugtupite, Watermelon Tourmaline. *Chakra:* heart, solar plexus

Feng Shui crystals: Ammolite (place crystals according to the bagua diagram on page 87 and see The Houses of

Life page 85)

career and life path: Ammolite, Anandalite, Azurite, Black Onyx, Black Tourmaline, Blue Calcite, Blue Jade, Blue Kyanite, Blue Tiger's Eye, Bumble Bee Jasper, Carnelian, Citrine, Clear Quartz, Goldstone, Green Aventurine, Hematite, Iron, Jet, Lapis Lazuli, Obsidian, Selenite, Shiva Shell, Smoky Quartz, Snowflake Obsidian, Sodalite, Stromatolite

children and creativity: Amethyst, Ammolite, Aquamarine, Black Tourmaline, Blue Chalcedony, Blue Lace Agate, Bumble Bee Jasper, Citrine, Golden Healer, Hematite, Ice Quartz, Jade, Labradorite, Milky Quartz, Moonstone, Opal, Optical Calcite, Rose Quartz, Specular Hematite Rose Quartz, Tiger's Eye, Triplite, Youngite

fame, reputation, status: Ammolite, Carnelian, Citrine, Clear Quartz, Fire Agate, Garnet, Gold, Herkimer Diamond, Kambaba Jasper, Purpurite, Red Jasper, Red Tiger's Eye, Ruby, Rutilated Quartz, Spirit Quartz, Sunstone

family and health: Amazonite, Amethyst, Ammolite, Apophyllite, Aventurine, Calcite, Celestite, Chrysocolla, Chrysoprase, Fluorite, Golden Healer, Jade, Malachite, Rhodochrosite, Rose Quartz, Smoky Quartz, Spirit Quartz

family/community: Amazonite, Chrysocolla, Green Calcite, Jade, Lapis Lazuli, Malachite, Rhyolite, Sodalite

front door for protection: Apache Tear, Black

Tourmaline, Hematite, Obsidian, Shungite

garden: Moss Agate, Quartz, Shungite

health/well-being: Apatite, Green Aventurine, Green Tourmaline, Jade, Petrified Wood, Pyrite, Shungite, Tiger's Eye

helpful people and travel: Ammolite, Anandalite, Brown Jade, Gold in Quartz, Jade, Malachite, Moonstone, Quartz, Quartz Cluster, Rutilated Quartz, Snow Quartz, Tourmalinated Quartz, Trigonic Quartz, Turquoise

home office or study: Amethyst, Ammolite, Fluorite, Jade, Pyrite, Sodalite

knowledge: Chrysocolla, Malachite with Azurite, Turquoise

love and relationships: Ammolite, Carnelian, Green Aventurine, Mangano Calcite, Menalite, Morganite, Pink Opal, Pink Tourmaline, Rhodochrosite, Rhodonite, Rose Quartz, Rose Quartz hearts and pink crystals, Shiva Lingam, Soulmate, Tiger's Eye

prosperity, wealth and abundance: Amethyst, Ammolite, Anandalite, Aventurine, Bloodstone, Chrysocolla, Citrine, Golden Herkimer, Goldstone, Jade and other green stones, Mookaite, Pyrite, Red Jasper, Serpentine, Unakite

skills and wisdom: Ammolite, Aventurine, Brandenberg, Clear Quartz, Fire and Ice, Selenite, cream or beige stones

spiritual well-being and heart: Amethyst, Ammolite, Carnelian, Citrine, Eye of the Storm, Herkimer

Diamond, Smoky Quartz

spirituality/personal growth: Amethyst, Apatite, Blue Lace Agate, Selenite

Firewall: Bismuth, Black Tourmaline, Eye of the Storm, Fire Agate, Galena (wash hands after use, make essence by indirect method), Labradorite, Master Shamanite, Mohawkite, Polychrome Jasper, Porcelain Jasper, Shungite, Stibnite, Tantalite, Titanite, Vanadinite (wash hands after use, make essence by indirect method). *Chakra:* higher heart

Forgiveness: Diopside, Green Aventurine, Khutnohorite, Mangano Calcite, Rose Quartz, Tugtupite. *Chakra:* higher heart

– G –

Gaia gateway chakra: Apache Tear, Basalt, Bastnasite, Black Actinolite, Black Calcite, Black Flint, Black Kyanite, Black Obsidian, Black Petalite, Black Spinel, Black Spot Herkimer Diamond, Day and Night Quartz, Fire and Ice, Granite, Jet, Master Shamanite, Mohawkite, Morion, Naturally Dark Smoky Quartz (not irradiated), Nebula Stone, Nirvana Quartz, Nuummite, Petalite, Preseli Bluestone, Sardonyx, Shungite, Smoky Elestial Quartz, Snowflake Obsidian, Specular Hematite, Spider Web Obsidian, Stromatolite, Tektite, Tibetan Black Spot Quartz, Tourmalinated Quartz, Verdelite. *Chakra:* below feet and/or on stellar gateway

> **balance and align:** Black Flint, Day and Night Quartz, Fire and Ice, Master Shamanite, Morion, Shungite, Tourmalinated Quartz, Verdelite

> **spin too rapid/stuck open:** Apache Tear, Basalt, Black Flint, Black Kyanite, Master Shamanite, Sardonyx, Shungite

> **spin too sluggish/stuck closed:** Black Spot Herkimer Diamond, Nirvana Quartz, Preseli Bluestone, Shungite, Specular Hematite, Tektite, Tibetan Black Spot Quartz

Geopathic stress: Amazonite, Amethyst, Black Tourmaline, Brown Jasper, Champagne Aura Quartz, Chlorite Quartz, Eye of the Storm, Flint, Gabbro, Granite, Graphic Smoky Quartz, Ironstone, Kunzite, Labradorite, Marble, Orgonite, Preseli Bluestone, Pyrite and

Sphalerite, Quartz, Riebekite with Sugilite and Bustamite, Selenite, Shieldite, Shungite, Smoky Amethyst, Smoky Elestial, Smoky Quartz, Sodalite, Tantalite, Tektite, Thunder Egg, Trummer Jasper. *Chakra:* earth star. Or place around corners of house.

Grounding: Ajo Quartz, Amphibole, Aztee, Banded Agate, Basalt, Blue Aragonite, Boji Stones, Bronzite, Brown Jasper, Bustamite, Calcite Fairy Stone, Champagne Aura Quartz, Chlorite Quartz, Cloudy Quartz, Dalmatian Stone, Empowerite, Fire Agate, Flint, Gabbro, Granite, Healer's Gold, Hematite, Hematoid Calcite, Herkimer Diamond, Honey Phantom Quartz, Kambaba Jasper, Keyiapo, Lazulite, Lemurian Jade, Lemurian Seed, Leopardskin Serpentine, Libyan Gold Tektite, Limonite, Luxullianite, Marcasite, Merlinite, Mohawkite, Novaculite, Nunderite, Peanut Wood, Pearl Spa Dolomite, Petrified Wood, Poppy Jasper, Preseli Bluestone, Purpurite, Pyrite in Magnesite, Quantum Quattro, Red Jasper, Rutile with Hematite, Schalenblende, Serpentine in Obsidian, Smoky Elestial Quartz, Smoky Herkimer, Smoky Quartz, Sodalite, Steatite, Stromatolite. *Chakra:* base, earth star, dantien

Group, containing your energies when in one: Black Tourmaline, Brown (Dravite) Tourmaline, Labradorite, Prehnite

Guru disconnection: Banded Agate, Rainbow Mayanite. *Chakra:* third eye, soma

– H –

Headache: Amber, Amblygonite, Azurite, Blue Sapphire, Bustamite, Cathedral Quartz, Champagne Aura Quartz, Dioptase, Dumortierite, Galena (wash hands after use, make essence by indirect method), Greenlandite, Hematite, Jet, Lapis Lazuli, Magnesite, Pyrite in Magnesite, Quantum Quattro, Rhodozite, Rose Quartz, Smoky Quartz, Sugilite, Turquoise. *Chakra:* third eye

> **from negative environmental factors/electromagnetic stress:** Galena (wash hands after use, make essence by indirect method), Smoky Quartz, Tektite

Health and well-being: see Feng Shui crystals (for the bagua) page 295

Heart chakra: Apophyllite, Aventurine, Chrysocolla, Chrysoprase, Cobalto Calcite, Danburite, Eudialyte, Gaia Stone, Green Jasper, Green Quartz, Green Sapphire, Green Siberian Quartz, Green Tourmaline, Hematite Quartz, Herkimer Diamond, Jade, Jadeite, Kunzite, Lavender Quartz, Lepidolite, Malachite, Morganite, Muscovite, Pink Danburite, Pink Petalite, Pink Tourmaline, Pyroxmangite, Red Calcite, Rhodochrosite, Rhodonite, Rhodozaz, Rose Quartz, Rubellite Tourmaline, Ruby, Ruby Lavender Quartz, Tugtupite, Variscite, Watermelon Tourmaline

> **balance and align:** Anandalite, Cobalto Calcite, Kunzite, Mangano Calcite, Ruby Lavender Quartz, Watermelon Tourmaline
>
> **clear heart chakra attachments:** Banded Agate,

Mangano Calcite

open the three-chambered heart: Danburite, Lemurian Aquitane Calcite, Mangano Calcite, Pink Petalite, Pink Tourmaline, Rosophia, Tugtupite

spin too rapid/stuck open: Green Tourmaline, Mangano Calcite, Quartz, Rose Quartz, Tugtupite

spin too sluggish/stuck closed: Calcite, Chohua Jasper, Danburite, Erythrite, Honey Calcite, Lemurian Jade, Pink Lemurian Seed, Red Calcite, Rhodozaz, Rose Quartz, Strawberry Quartz, Tugtupite

Heart, physical: Adamite, Andean Blue Opal, Brandenberg Amethyst, Bustamite, Cacoxenite, Candle Quartz, Fiskenaesset Ruby, Garnet in Quartz, Golden Danburite, Golden Healer, Green Aventurine, Green Diopside, Green Heulandite, Holly Agate, Khutnohorite, Merlinite, Picrolite, Prasiolite, Quantum Quattro, Rhodochrosite, Rhodonite, Rose Elestial Quartz, Rose Quartz, Rosophia, Tugtupite. *Chakra:* heart

Heart seed chakra: Ajo Blue Calcite, Ajoite, Azeztulite, Brandenberg Amethyst, Coral, Danburite, Dianite, Fire Opal, Golden Healer, Green Ridge Quartz, Khutnohorite, Lemurian Calcite, Lilac Quartz, Macedonian Opal, Mangano Calcite, Merkabite Calcite, Pink Opal, Pyroxmangite, Rhodozaz, Roselite, Rosophia, Ruby Lavender Quartz, Scolecite, Spirit Quartz, Tugtupite, Violane. Place at base of breastbone.

balance and align: Danburite, Golden Healer, Golden Herkimer, Khutnohorite, Merkabite Calcite

spin too rapid/stuck open: Ajo Blue Calcite,

Khutnohorite, Macedonian Opal

spin too sluggish/stuck closed: Fire Opal, Rhodozaz, Rosophia, Spirit Quartz

Helplessness: Actinolite Quartz, Adamite, Brazilianite, Bronzite, Clevelandite, Covellite, Dumortierite, Kakortokite, Mystic Topaz, Ocean Jasper, Paraiba Tourmaline, Pumice, Quantum Quattro, Sceptre Quartz, Tree Agate. *Chakra:* earth star, base, sacral, dantien

High frequency communication aerials, microwaves, infrared and radar: Amazonite, Amethyst, Black Moonstone, Black Tourmaline, Chlorite Quartz, Fluorite, Gabbro, Germanium, Granite, Graphic Smoky Quartz, Hematite, Herkimer Diamond, Klinoptilolith, Malachite, Orgonite, Reinerite, Shieldite, Shungite, Smoky Elestial Quartz, Smoky Quartz, Sodalite, Sphalerite, Tourmalinated Quartz, Tourmaline, Yellow Kunzite, Zeolite. Place around site or between you and the site.

Higher heart chakra: Ajo Blue Calcite, Amazonite, Anandalite (Aurora Quartz), Aqua Aura Quartz, Azeztulite, Bloodstone, Celestite, Danburite, Dioptase, Dream Quartz, Eye of the Storm, Fire and Ice Quartz, Gaia Stone, Green Siberian Quartz, Khutnohorite, Kunzite, Lavender Quartz, Lazurine, Lilac Quartz, Macedonian Opal, Mangano Calcite, Muscovite, Nirvana Quartz, Phenacite, Pink Crackle Quartz, Pink Lazurine, Pink or Lilac Danburite, Pink Petalite, Pyroxmangite, Quantum Quattro, Que Sera, Rainbow Mayanite, Raspberry Aura Quartz, Rhodozaz, Rose Opal, Rose Elestial Quartz, Rose Quartz, Roselite, Rosophia, Ruby

Aura Quartz, Ruby Lavender Quartz™, Spirit Quartz, Strawberry Lemurian, Strawberry Quartz, Tangerose, Tugtupite, Turquoise. *Chakra:* higher heart

> **balance and align:** Bloodstone, Eye of the Storm, Quantum Quattro, Que Sera, Tangerose
>
> **spin too rapid/stuck open:** Eye of the Storm, Mangano Calcite, Pink Petalite, Rose Elestial Quartz, Turquoise
>
> **spin too sluggish/stuck closed:** Quantum Quattro, Que Sera, Ruby Aura Quartz, Strawberry Lemurian

Higher self, contact: Amphibole, Anandalite, Anthrophyllite, Azeztulite, Brandenberg, Bushman Red Cascade Quartz, Cathedral Quartz, Celtic Quartz, Danburite, Elestial Quartz, Faden Quartz, Fire and Ice Quartz, Golden Healer Quartz, Green Ridge Quartz, Mangano Vesuvianite, Orange River Quartz, Petalite, Porphyrite (Chinese Letter Stone), Prasiolite, Rose Quartz, Rosophia, Sugar Blade Quartz, Trigonic Quartz, Ussingite

Home/other buildings, protection: Black Tourmaline, Dravide Tourmaline, Halite, Hanksite, Holey Stones, Malachite, Quartz, Rose Quartz, Ruby, Sardonyx, Selenite, Witches Finger

'Hooks', remove: Aventurine, Charoite, Drusy Golden Healer, Flint, Goethite, Green Aventurine, Klinoptilolith, Nunderite, Orange Kyanite, Pyromorphite, Rainbow Mayanite, Stibnite, Tantalite. *Chakra:* sacral, solar plexus, third eye

Ill wishing, protection against: Actinolite, Amethyst, Black Tourmaline, Blue Chalcedony, Bronzite (use with caution as may amplify), Crackled Fire Agate, Fire Agate, Galena (caution, potentially toxic), Limonite, Master Shamanite, Mohawkite, Nunderite, Nuummite, Purpurite, Richterite, Rose Quartz, Tantalite, Tugtupite. *Chakra:* throat (wear continuously)

Ill wishing, return to source so that effect is understood: Beryl, Bronzite, Calcite, Chalcedony, Quartz, Selenite, Silver

Illusions, dispel: Adularia, Fairy Wand Quartz, Ilmenite, Lemurian Seed, Lepidocrocite, Kornerupine, Neptunite, Nirvana Quartz, Quartz with Mica, Vivianite

Immune system: Agate, Amechlorite, Ametrine, Anandalite™, Black or Green Tourmaline, Bloodstone, Blue Agate, Brown Jasper, Carnelian, Chevron Amethyst, Chiastolite, Chohua Jasper, Diaspore (Zultanite), Emerald, Fuchsite, Fuchsite with Ruby, Green Calcite, Klinoptilolith, Kunzite, Lapis Lazuli, Lemurian Jade, Lepidolite, Macedonian Green Opal, Malachite (use as polished stone, make essence by indirect method), Mookaite Jasper, Moss Agate, Nzuri Moyo, Ocean Jasper, Paraiba Tourmaline, Pentagonite, Petrified Wood, Preseli Bluestone, Quantum Quattro, Quartz, Que Sera, Reinerite, Richterite, Rosophia, Ruby in Zoisite, Schalenblende, Seriphos Quartz, Shungite, Smithsonite, Smoky Quartz with Aegerine, Super 7, Tangerose,

Thunder Egg, Titanite (Sphene), Tourmaline, Turquoise, Winchite, Zoisite. *Chakra:* dantien, higher heart. Place around corners of bed.

Implants, remove: Ajoite, Amechlorite, Cryolite, Drusy Golden Healer, Green Aventurine, Holly Agate, Ilmenite, Lemurian Aquitane Calcite, Lemurian Seed, Novaculite, Nuummite, Rainbow Mayanite, Stibnite, Tantalite. *Chakra:* crown

Incarnation, ameliorate discomfort in: Ajo Blue Calcite, Celestobarite, Empowerite, Golden Healer, Guardian Stone, Keyiapo, Orange Kyanite, Peanut Wood, Pearl Spar Dolomite, Polychrome Jasper, Red Celestial Quartz, Riebekite with Sugilite and Bustamite, Rosophia, Sanda Rosa Azeztulite, Snakeskin Agate, Strontianite, Thompsonite. *Chakra:* soma, dantien and earth star

Inferiority complex: Pyrite in Magnesite. *Chakra:* dantien

Injuries, past life: Brandenberg Amethyst, Herkimer Diamond, Onyx. *Chakra:* past life, causal vortex

Injury, protection against: Tourmaline, Turquoise

Inner child: Cobalto Calcite, Dalmatian Stone, Fairy Quartz, Golden Healer, Hanksite, Limonite, Pink Crackle Quartz, Quantum Quattro, Spirit Quartz, Voegesite, Youngite. *Chakra:* sacral

Inner critic: Aventurine, Blue Chalcedony, Freedom Stone, Rainbow Obsidian, Rose Quartz, Rutilated Quartz

Insomnia: Ajoite, Ajoite with Shattuckite, Amethyst, Bloodstone, Candle Quartz, Celestite, Charoite, Glendonite, Hematite, Howlite, Khutnohorite, Lapis Lazuli, Lepidolite, Magnetite (Lodestone) (place at head and foot of bed), Moonstone, Mount Shasta Opal, Muscovite, Ocean Jasper, Petrified Wood, Pink Sunstone, Poldervaarite, Rosophia, Selenite, Shungite, Sodalite, Tektite, Topaz, Zoisite. Place by the bed or under the pillow.

disturbed sleep patterns: Khutnohorite, Ocean Jasper, Owyhee Blue Opal, Petrified Wood, Sodalite

from geopathic/electromagnetic stress/pollution: Black Tourmaline, Chlorite Quartz, Crystal Cap Amethyst, Eye of the Storm, Gabbro, Guinea Fowl Jasper, Herkimer Diamond, Klinoptilolith, Labradorite, Marble, Ocean Jasper, Orgonite, Red Amethyst, Shieldite, Shungite, Smoky Herkimer Diamond, Smoky Quartz, Sodalite, Spectrolite, Tektite, Thunder Egg. Place around bed and/or around the four corners of the room or house, depending on how strong the stress.

negative environmental influences: Black Tourmaline, Bloodstone, Champagne Aura Quartz, Klinoptilolith, Lepidolite, Marble, Orgonite, Shungite, Smoky Elestial Quartz, Smoky Quartz, Tantalite, Trummer Jasper, Turquoise. Place around the four corners of the room.

nightmares/night terrors: Dalmatian Stone, Fairy Quartz, Smoky Quartz, Sodalite, Spirit Quartz, Tourmaline, Tremolite. *Chakra:* third eye

overactive mind: Amethyst, Auralite 23, Blue Selenite, Bytownite (Yellow Labradorite), Crystal Cap Amethyst, Rhodozite, Sodalite, Spectrolite. *Chakra:*

third eye

stress: Amethyst, Chrysoprase, Eye of the Storm, Lemurian Gold Opal, Riebekite with Sugilite and Bustamite, Rose Quartz, Shungite, Sodalite, Tektite. *Chakra:* higher heart

Intention, support: Brandenberg, Desert Rose, Iron Pyrite, Manifestation Crystal (a crystal that has a smaller crystal completely contained within it), Phantom Quartz, Rose Quartz, Topaz, Watermelon Tourmaline

Interface, create between self and outside world: Andescine Labradorite, Brochantite, Green Aventurine, Green Fluorite, Healer's Gold, Iridescent Pyrite, Jade, Labradorite, Lemurian Jade, Master Shamanite, Mohawkite, Nunderite, Richterite, Scheelite, Serpentine in Obsidian, Spectrolite, Tantalite. *Chakra:* spleen, dantien

Irritant filter: Halite, Limestone, Pumice, Rhodochrosite, Shungite. *Chakra:* dantien

– J –

Jealousy: Eclipse Stone, Green Aventurine, Heulandite, Mangano Calcite, Rainbow Mayanite, Rose Quartz, Rosophia, Tugtupite, Zircon. *Chakra:* heart
Jetlag: Preseli Bluestone, Shungite

– K –

Karmic cleansing: Cloudy Quartz, Flint, Golden Healer, Holly Agate, Lemurian Seed, Wind Fossil Agate. *Chakra:* past life
Karmic/ancestral contracts: Ancestralite, Boli Stone, Cradle of Humankind, Freedom Stone, Gabbro, Leopardskin Jasper, Phantom Quartz, Red Amethyst, Wind Fossil Agate. *Chakra:* past life, causal vortex
Karmic debris: Golden Healer, Nuummite, Peach Selenite, Rainbow Mayanite, Smoky Spirit Quartz, Wind Fossil Agate. *Chakra:* past life
Karmic debts, release: Ancestralite, Freedom Stone, Holly Agate, Nuummite. *Chakra:* past life
Karmic dis-ease: Covellite, Dumortierite, Golden Healer, Isis Calcite, Kambaba Jasper, Nuummite, Stromatolite, and see Past Life page 319. *Chakra:* past life
Karmic/ancestral   enmeshment/entanglements: Ancestralite, Blue Flint, Freedom Stone, Golden Healer, Green Aventurine, Novaculite, Nuummite, Peach Selenite, Rainbow Mayanite, Smoky Elestial Quartz. *Chakra:* past life, causal vortex

Karmic wounds: Ajo Quartz, Ajoite, Dumortierite, Golden Healer, Green Ridge Quartz, Lemurian Seed, Macedonian Opal, Mookaite Jasper, Rathbunite™, Rosophia, Scheelite, Xenotine

– L –

Learning from past lives: Ancestralite, Lakelandite, Muscovite, Peridot. *Chakra:* past life, causal vortex

Letting go of past: Axinite, Fenster Quartz, Flint, Fulgarite, Green Diopside, Kakortokite, Kimberlite, Lepidocrocite, Nuummite, Paraiba Tourmaline, Pumice, Scheelite, Zircon. *Chakra:* solar plexus, heart, past life

Limiting patterns of behaviour: Ajoite, Amphibole, Arfvedsonite, Atlantasite, Barite, Botswana Agate, Bronzite, Cassiterite, Celadonite, Chlorite Shaman Quartz, Crackled Fire Agate, Dalmatian Stone, Datolite, Dream Quartz, Dumortierite, Epidote, Garnet in Quartz, Glendonite, Halite, Hanksite, Hematoid Calcite, Honey Phantom Calcite, Indicolite Quartz, Kinoite, Marcasite, Merlinite, Nuummite, Oligocrase, Owyhee Blue Opal, Pearl Spa Dolomite, Porphyrite (Chinese Letter Stone), Quantum Quattro, Rainbow Covellite, Scheelite, Spider Web Obsidian, Stellar Beam Calcite. *Chakra:* base, sacral, dantien, solar plexus, past life

Love, compassionate: Bixbite, Candle Quartz, Mangano Vesuvianite, Rose Quartz, Tugtupite

Love, old, cut the cords of: Flint, Green Aventurine, Lemurian Aquitane Calcite, Novaculite, Nunderite, Nuummite, Rainbow Mayanite, Rainbow Obsidian. *Chakra:* solar plexus, sacral, past life, spleen, heart

Love, unconditional: Cobalto Calcite, Crystalline Kyanite, Gaia Stone, Lemurian Seed, Poldervaarite, Rose Aura Quartz, Rose Quartz, Smoky Rose Quartz,

Tangerine Aura, Tiffany Stone, Tugtupite, Zircon. *Chakra:* higher heart

– M –

ME: Ametrine, Bismuth, Chinese Red Quartz, Chrysolite in Serpentine, Eye of the Storm, Petrified Wood, Quantum Quattro, Que Sera, Ruby, Shungite, Tourmaline. *Chakra:* dantien, higher heart

Memory, improve: Amber, Amethyst, Barite, Coprolite, Emerald, Fluorite, Hematoid Calcite, Herderite, Klinoptilolith, Marcasite, Moss Agate, Opal, Phantom Calcite, Pyrite and Sphalerite, Pyrolusite, Rhodonite, Unakite, Vivianite. *Chakra:* third eye, crown

Memory, release suppressed: Cradle of Humankind, Freedom Stone, Revelation Stone

Mental abuse: Apricot Quartz, Golden Healer, Lazurine, Proustite, Tugtupite with Nuummite, Yellow Crackle Quartz, Xenotine

Mental attachments: Aegerine, Banded Agate, Blue Halite, Limonite, Pyrolusite, Smoky Amethyst, Yellow Phantom Quartz. *Chakra:* third eye

Mental conditioning, rigid: Drusy Golden Healer, Pholocomite, Rainbow Covellite, and see Neurotic patterns page 316. *Chakra:* third eye, crown

Mental detox: Amechlorite, Banded Agate, Drusy Quartz on Sphalerite, Eye of the Storm, Golden Healer, Larvikite, Pyrite in Magnesite, Rainbow Covellite, Richterite, Shungite, Smoky Quartz with Aegerine, Spirit Quartz, Tantalite

Mental imperatives, release: Danburite, Idocrase. *Chakra*: past life, soma

Mental implants: Amechlorite, Blue Halite, Brandenberg, Cryolite, Drusy Golden Healer, Holly Agate, Ilmenite, Lemurian Aquitane Calcite, Novaculite, Nuummite, Pholocomite, Tantalite

Mental possession: Aegerine

Mental sabotage: Agrellite, Amphibole, Lemurian Aquitane Calcite, Mohawkite, Paraiba Tourmaline, Tantalite, Yellow Scapolite

Mental undue influence, remove: Banded Agate, Limonite, Novaculite, Tantalite

Metabolic imbalances: Amazonite, Amechlorite, Azurite with Malachite and Chrysocolla (use as polished stone, make essence by indirect method), Blue Opal, Bornite, Champagne Aura Quartz, Chrysocolla, Diamond, Galaxyite, Garnet, Golden Azeztulite, Golden Danburite, Golden Herkimer, Hackmanite, Healer's Gold, Herkimer Diamond, Khutnohorite, Labradorite, Lemurian Jade, Mangano Vesuvianite, Peridot, Quantum Quattro, Que Sera, Shungite, Sonora Sunrise, Tantalite, Tanzine Aura Quartz, Tugtupite, Watermelon Tourmaline, Winchite. *Chakra:* dantien, third eye

Microwaves: Amazonite, Amethyst, Black Moonstone, Black Tourmaline, Chlorite Quartz, Fluorite, Gabbro, Germanium, Granite, Graphic Smoky Quartz, Hematite, Herkimer Diamond, Klinoptilolith, Malachite, Orgonite, Reinerite, Shieldite, Shungite, Smoky Elestial Quartz, Smoky Quartz, Sodalite, Sphalerite, Tourmalinated Quartz, Tourmaline, Yellow Kunzite, Zeolite. Place around site or between you and the site.

Multidimensional cellular healing: Ajo Blue Calcite, Ajo Quartz, Anandalite™, Annabergite, Brandenberg Amethyst, Crystal Cap Amethyst, Elestial Quartz, Eudialyte, Fire and Ice Quartz, Fiskenaesset Ruby, Golden Coracalcite, Golden Healer Quartz, Mangano Vesuvianite, Messina Quartz, Pollucite, Que Sera, Rhodozite, Ruby Lavender Quartz

Multidimensional soul healing: Ajo Quartz, Anandalite™, Banded Agate, Celestobarite, Celtic Healer, Eudialyte, Fiskenaesset Ruby, Golden Healer, Halite, Hanksite, Icicle Calcite, Kakortokite, Lemurian Seed, Lilac Quartz, Phantom Quartz, Que Sera, Rutile with Hematite, Sanda Rosa Azeztulite, Satyamani and Satyaloka Quartz, Shaman Quartz, Sichuan Quartz, Spirit Quartz, Tangerine Dream Lemurian, Trigonic Quartz

Multidimensional travel: Afghanite, Anandalite™, Auralite 23, Aztee, Banded Agate, Blue Moonstone, Brandenberg Amethyst, Celestobarite, Celtic Quartz, Golden Selenite, Kinoite, Novaculite, Nunderite, Orange Creedite, Owyhee Blue Opal, Phantom Quartz, Polychrome Jasper, Preseli Bluestone, Rainbow Moonstone, Sedona Stone, Shaman Quartz, Spectrolite, Spirit Quartz, Tanzanite, Thunder Egg, Titanite (Sphene), Trigonic Quartz, Ussingite, Vivianite, Youngite

– N –

Necessary change, accept: Axinite, Eclipse Stone, Ethiopian Opal, Luxullianite, Nunderite, Snakeskin Pyrite. *Chakra:* dantien

Negative energies, protection from: Amethyst, Apache Tear, Black Kyanite, Black Obsidian, Black Onyx, Black Tourmaline, Bornite, Celestite, Citrine, Elestial Quartz, Eye of the Storm, Hematite, Jet, Katanganite, Kunzite, Labradorite, Peacock Ore, Plancheite, Shungite, Smoky Quartz, Ussingite

Negative energy, dispel: Apache Tear, Black Kyanite, Golden Healer, Guardian Stone, Hypersthene, Klinoptilolith, Nuummite, Pumice, Smoky Elestial Quartz, Smoky Herkimer, Tantalite. *Chakra:* throat, earth star

Negative energy, transmute: Amber, Amethyst, Black Tourmaline, Heulandite, Lapis Lazuli, Pollucite, Pumice, Orgonite, Scolecite, Shungite, Smoky Quartz, Snowflake Obsidian, Sodalite, Stilbite, Thompsonite, and see Detoxification page 281

Negative ions, increase: Amber, Amethyst, Angel's Wing Calcite, Bismuth, Germanium, Halite, Heulandite, Jasper, Klinoptilolith, Lepidolite, Pollucite, Orgonite, Quartz, Renierite, Rubellite, Scolecite, Shungite, Sphalerite, Stilbite, Thompsonite, Tourmaline

Negative karma release: Smoky Elestial Quartz, and see Past life page 319. *Chakra:* past life

Neurotic patterns: Arfvedsonite, Celadonite, Greenlandite,

Porphyrite (Chinese Letter Stone), Rainbow Covellite, Scheelite. *Chakra:* solar plexus

Nightmares/night terrors: Amethyst, Celestite, Chrysoprase, Dalmatian Stone, Diaspore, Hematite, Jet, Mangano Calcite, Pearl Spa Dolomite, Prehnite, Rose Quartz, Ruby, Smoky Quartz, Sodalite, Spirit Quartz, Tremolite, Turquoise. Place under the pillow or around the bed.

Nuclear sites, transmute radiation effects: Amber, Aventurine, Boron, Chlorite Quartz, Colemanite, Covellite, Galena (wash hands after use, make essence by indirect method), Graphic Smoky Quartz, Hackmanite, Kernite, Larimar, Lepidolite, Libyan Gold Tektite, Malachite, Malacolla, Mica, Morion, Orgonite, Rainbow Covellite, Shungite, Smoky Elestial Quartz, Smoky Quartz, Sodalite, Tantalite, Tektite, Torbernite, Velvet Malachite. Place stones around site or between you and the source.

– O –

Obsession: Ammolite, Auralite 23, Barite, Bytownite, Fenster Quartz, Golden Selenite, Novaculite, Nuummite, Ocean Jasper, Red Amethyst, Spirit Quartz, Tantalite, Vera Cruz Amethyst. *Chakra:* dantien, solar plexus, third eye

Obsessive behaviour: Ocean Jasper, Smoky Rose Quartz, Tantalite

Obsessive thoughts: Ammolite, Auralite 23, Barite, Bytownite, Fluorite, Optical Calcite, Rhomboid Selenite, Scolecite, Spirit Quartz, Tantalite. *Chakra:* third eye, crown

Obsessive-compulsive disorder: Amethyst Herkimer, Fenster Quartz, Flint, Novaculite, Tantalite

Oppression: Blizzard Stone

Other people's thoughts invading: Amethyst, Auralite 23, Black Tourmaline, Fluorite, Labradorite, Shamanite. *Chakra:* third eye

Outworn patterns: Amphibole, Arfvedsonite, Brandenberg Amethyst, Celadonite, Garnet in Quartz, Owyhee Blue Opal, Porphyrite (Chinese Letter Stone), Quantum Quattro, Rainbow Covellite, Rainbow Mayanite, Scheelite, Stibnite. *Chakra:* earth star, base, sacral, solar plexus, third eye

Over-attachment: Drusy Golden Healer, Rainbow Mayanite, Tantalite, Tinguaite. *Chakra:* solar plexus

Overwhelm: Diopside. *Chakra:* solar plexus

– P –

Palm chakra: Golden Healer, Spangolite. *Chakra:* palm
Palm chakra, too open: Flint, Labradorite
Panic attacks: Amethyst, Blue-green Smithsonite, Dumortierite, Eye of the Storm, Girasol, Green Phantom Quartz, Green Tourmaline, Kunzite, Serpentine in Obsidian, Tremolite, Turquoise. *Chakra:* heart, higher heart, solar plexus. Keep in pocket and hold when required.
Past life/ancestral conflict, resolve: Ancestralite, Bixbite, Champagne Aura Quartz, Cradle of Humankind, Fluorapatite, Freedom Stone, Purpurite, Rainbow Mayanite, Trigonic Quartz
Past life/ancestral debts, recognize: Lemurian Seed, Nuummite, Okenite, Purple Scapolite. *Chakra:* past life, solar plexus
Past life/ancestral healing: Ancestralite, Blizzard Stone, Charoite, Chinese Red Quartz, Cradle of Humankind, Danburite, Dumortierite, Garnet in Quartz, Golden Healer, Infinite Stone, Lakelandite, Lodolite, Merlinite, Obsidian, Okenite, Oregon Opal, Peanut Wood, Picasso Jasper, Pietersite, Rhodonite, Serpentine in Obsidian, Tanzanite, Tibetan Quartz, Tugtupite, Voegesite. *Chakra:* past life
Past life chakras: Ammolite, Astraline, Black Moonstone, Blizzard Stone, Brandenberg Amethyst, Catlinite, Chrysotile in Serpentine, Coprolite, Cuprite with Chrysocolla, Dinosaur Bone, Dumortierite, Ethiopian

Opal, Fire and Ice, Flint, Keyiapo, Larvikite, Lemurian Aquatine Calcite, Madagascar Quartz, Mystic Merlinite, Nuummite, Oceanite (Blue Onyx), Oregon Opal, Peanut Wood, Petrified Wood, Preseli Bluestone, Rainbow Mayanite, Rainbow Moonstone, Reinerite, Rhodozite, Rhyolite, Scheelite, Serpentine in Obsidian, Shiva Lingam, Smoky Amethyst, Tangerose, Tantalite, Titanite, Variscite, Violane (Blue Dioptase), Voegesite, Wind Fossil Agate

> **balance and align:** Dumortierite, Picasso Jasper, Rainbow Mayanite, Tangerose, Titanite, Violane (Blue Dioptase)
>
> **spin too rapid/stuck open:** Black Moonstone, Coprolite, Flint, Petrified Wood, Preseli Bluestone, Scheelite, Sea Sediment Jasper, Tantalite
>
> **spin too sluggish/stuck closed:** Blizzard Stone, Dragon Stone, Dumortierite, Garnet in Quartz, Rhodozite, Serpentine in Obsidian, Tantalite

Past life cord cutting: Charoite, Flint, Green Aventurine, Green Obsidian, Malachite, Novaculite, Nuummite, Petalite, Rainbow Mayanite, Rainbow Obsidian, Smoky Amethyst, Sunstone, Wulfenite. *Chakra:* past life, base, sacral, solar plexus, third eye

Past life dis-ease: Celtic Quartz, Dumortierite, Golden Healer, Lemurian Seed, Sichuan Quartz, Tanzanite with Iolite and Danburite. *Chakra:* past life, causal vortex

Past life effect on present: Rhodozite

Past life entity attachment: Chrysotile in Serpentine, Drusy Golden Healer, Green Aventurine, Ilmenite,

Larvikite, Lemurian Aquitane Calcite, Novaculite, Nuummite, Pyromorphite, Quantum Quattro, Rainbow Mayanite, Smoky Amethyst, Stibnite, Tantalite, Tinguaite, Tugtupite, Valentinite and Stibnite. *Chakra:* past life, sacral, solar plexus, spleen, third eye

Past life imperatives, release: Ammolite, Lemurian Aquitane Calcite, Novaculite, Nuummite, Tantalite

Past life implants: Amechlorite, Chlorite Quartz, Cryolite, Drusy Golden Healer, Green Aventurine, Holly Agate, Ilmenite, Lemurian Aquitane Calcite, Novaculite, Nuummite, Rainbow Mayanite, Stibnite, Tantalite, Tinguaite

Past life injuries: Flint, Golden Healer, Herkimer Diamond, Onyx. *Chakra:* past life

Past life jealousies: Rainbow Mayanite, Rose Quartz

Past life manipulation: Nuummite, Tantalite

Past life mental imperatives, release: Danburite, Golden Danburite, Golden Healer, Idocrase, Nuummite, Septarian, Tantalite. *Chakra:* past life

Past life misuse of power: Nuummite, Ocean Jasper, Sceptre Quartz, Smoky Lemurian Seed

Past life, phobias resulting from: Carolite, Dumortierite, Golden Healer, Oceanite, Prehnite, Serpentine in Obsidian. *Chakra:* past life

Past life soul agreements: Brandenberg Amethyst, Green Ridge Quartz, Nuummite, Trigonic Quartz, Wind Fossil Agate, Wulfenite. *Chakra:* past life, higher crown

Past life, soul loss resulting from: Chrysotile in Serpentine, Fulgarite

Past life thought forms, release: Aegerine, Auralite 23, Iolite, Pyromorphite, Scolecite, Septarian, Spectrolite, Xenotine. *Chakra:* past life, third eye

Past life trauma: Blue Euclase, Brandenberg Amethyst, Dumortierite, Empowerite, Golden Healer, Mangano Vesuvianite, Oceanite, Oregon Opal, Phantom Crystals, Red Phantom Quartz, Ruby Lavender Quartz, Smoky Elestial Quartz, Smoky Herkimer, Tantalite, Victorite. *Chakra:* past life, causal vortex

Past life vows: Blue Aventurine, Nuummite, Rainbow Mayanite, Stibnite, Wind Fossil Agate. *Chakra:* past life, third eye

Past life wound imprints in etheric body: Ajo Quartz, Anandalite, Brandenberg Amethyst, Charoite, Diaspore (Zultanite), Ethiopian Opal, Eye of the Storm, Flint, Golden Healer, Green Ridge Quartz, Lemurian Aquitane Calcite, Lemurian Seed, Macedonian Opal, Master Shamanite, Mookaite Jasper, Rainbow Mayanite, Sceptre Quartz, Selenite, Smoky Quartz, Snakeskin Pyrite, Stibnite, Tantalite, Tibetan Black Spot Quartz. *Chakra:* past life, causal vortex. Or place over site.

Past lives, access: Brandenberg Amethyst, Cavansite, Chrysotile, Cradle of Humankind, Dream Quartz, Dumortierite, Faden Quartz, Fiskenaesset Ruby, Lemurian Seed, Nuummite, Oregon Opal, Preseli Bluestone, Trigonic Quartz. *Chakra:* past life, third eye, causal vortex

Past, release from: Dumortierite, Elestial Quartz, Smoky Amethyst, and see Past lives above. *Chakra:* past life, earth star, base

Personal power, regain: Basalt, Brandenberg Amethyst, Conichalcite, Empowerite, Eudialyte, Eye of the Storm, Kundalini Quartz, Orange Kyanite, Owyhee Blue Opal, Sedona Stone, Shungite, Tinguaite, Triplite. *Chakra:* base, dantien

Physical protection: Agate, Amethyst, Apache Tear, Black Tourmaline, Carnelian, Fluorite, Labradorite, Master Shamanite, Mohawkite, Peridot, Sard, Smoky Quartz, Tantalite, Turquoise, Zircon

Poison, protect against: Amethyst, Diamond, Fluorite, Serpentine

Polarization (realign to Earth's magnetic field): Aragonite, Eye of the Storm, Labradorite, Magnesite, Preseli Bluestone

Pollutants, anti: Amazonite, Amber, Amethyst, Aventurine, Black Tourmaline, Blue Sapphire, Brown Jasper, Chlorite Quartz, Halite, Hanksite, Larimar, Malachite, Opal, Orgonite, Purple Tourmaline, Quantum Quattro, Shieldite, Shungite, Smoky Quartz, Sodalite, Turquoise. *Chakra:* earth star. Place stones in environment to absorb.

Positive ions, decrease: see Negative ions, increase page 316

Possessions, protect: Ruby, Sardonyx, Zircon

Pregnancy and childbirth, protect during: Ammolite, Ammonite, Chrysocolla, Eye of the Storm, Geodes, Hematite, Lepidolite, Malachite, Menalite, Moonstone, Picture Jasper, Rose Quartz

Prohibitions on using psychic sight, undo: Apophyllite pyramid, Aquamarine, Astrophyllite, Azurite, Bytownite, Lapis Lazuli, Rhomboid Selenite. *Chakra:* third eye

Protection against radiation: Amber, Malachite, Rutilated Quartz, Smoky Quartz, Star Sapphire

Protection, angelic: Amethyst, Angelite, Angel's Wing Calcite, Celestite, Selenite, Seraphinite

Protection, aura: see Aura page 262

Protection, children: Agate, Bloodstone, Blue Lace Agate, Carnelian, Green Moss Agate, Jade, Ruby, Youngite. Wear constantly.

Protection, during astral travel: Brecciated Jasper, Kyanite, Leopardskin Agate, Preseli Bluestone, Red Jasper, Shaman Quartz, Snakeskin Agate, Stibnite, Yellow Jasper, and see Travel, shamanic journeys page 347

Protection, from crime and/or violence: Jet, Sardonyx, Selenite, Turquoise

Protection, from negative energies: Amethyst, Apache Tear, Black Kyanite, Black Obsidian, Black Onyx, Black Tourmaline, Bornite, Celestite, Chalcopyrite, Citrine, Elestial Quartz, Eye of the Storm, Flint, Jet, Kunzite, Plancheite, Quartz, Rose Quartz, Selenite, Shungite, Smoky Quartz. Wear or grid around home or environment.

Protection, general: Agate, Amber, Apache Tear, Aventurine, Banded Agate, Beryl, Black Kyanite, Black Obsidian, Black Tourmaline, Boji Stones, Bronzite, Calcite, Carnelian, Cat's Eye, Chalcedony, Chiastolite,

Chrysoprase, Citrine, Dravite Tourmaline, Emerald, Fire Agate, Fire Opal, Flint, Fluorite, Golden Topaz, Halite, Hanksite, Heliodor (Golden Beryl), Hematite, Hematoid Quartz, Herkimer Diamond, Holey Stones, Honey Calcite, Imperial Topaz, Jade, Jasper, Jet, Labradorite, Lapis Lazuli, Lepidolite, Magnesite (Lodestone), Mahogany Obsidian, Malachite, Marble, Mookaite Jasper, Moss Agate, Nuummite, Ocean Jasper, Peridot, Petrified Wood, Polychrome Jasper, Prehnite, Pumice, Pyrite, Quartz, Red Jasper, Ruby, Rutilated Quartz, Sapphire, Sard, Sardonyx, Selenite, Serpentine, Shungite, Snowflake Obsidian, Staurolite, Sulphur, Sunstone, Tiger's Eye, Topaz, Tourmaline, Tourmalinated Quartz, Tree Agate, Turquoise, Turritella Agate, Yellow Jasper, Zircon

Protection, home, other buildings: see Home page 304

Protection, possessions: Ruby, Sardonyx, Zircon

Protection, pregnancy and childbirth: see Pregnancy page 323

Protection, travel: see Travel page 346

Psychic attack, protect against: Black Tourmaline, Brandenburg Amethyst, Labradorite, Master Shamanite, Mohawkite, Nunderite, Nuummite, Polychrome Jasper, Richterite, Shungite, Tantalite, Tugtupite. Wear constantly. *Chakra:* throat, higher heart

Psychic blockages, remove: Afghanite, Ajo Quartz, Blue Selenite, Bytownite, Rainbow Mayanite, Rhodozite, Rhomboid Selenite

Psychic implants/imprints: Amechlorite, Brandenberg

Amethyst, Cryolite, Drusy Golden Healer, Ethiopian Opal, Flint, Holly Agate, Ilmenite, Lemurian Aquitane Calcite, Novaculite, Nuummite, Pyromorphite, Rainbow Mayanite, Snakeskin Pyrite, Stichtite, Tantalite

Psychic interference, block: Afghanite, Black Tourmaline, Labradorite, Master Shamanite, Nuummite, Purpurite, Rainbow Mayanite, Shungite, Tantalite. *Chakra:* throat and third eye

Psychic manipulation: Nuummite

Psychic mugging: Tugtupite. *Chakra:* higher heart

Psychic overwhelm: Limonite, Master Shamanite

Psychic protection: Amber, Amethyst, Ancestralite, Angelite, Apache Tear, Aventurine, Black Moonstone, Black Obsidian, Black Tourmaline, Bronzite, Chlorite Quartz, Eye of the Storm, Fluorite, Jade, Jet, Labradorite, Lapis Lazuli, Lemurian Seed Crystal, Master Shamanite, Mohawkite, Moqui Marbles, Nuummite, Petalite, Prehnite, Pyrite, Ruby, Seraphinite, Stibnite, Sugilite, Tantalite, Tiger Iron, Tiger's Eye, and see Psychic attack, above.

Psychic shield: Actinolite, Amphibole, Azotic Topaz, Aztee, Black Tourmaline, Bornite, Bowenite (New Jade), Brandenberg Amethyst, Brazilianite, Celestobarite, Chlorite Shaman Quartz, Crackled Fire Agate, Eye of the Storm, Fiskenaesset Ruby, Frondellite with Strengite, Gabbro, Graphic Smoky Quartz (Zebra Stone), Hanksite, Iridescent Pyrite, Keyiapo, Labradorite, Lorenzenite (Ramsayite), Marcasite, Master Shamanite, Mohave Turquoise, Mohawkite, Owyhee Blue Opal, Polychrome

Jasper, Purpurite, Pyromorphite, Quantum Quattro, Red Amethyst, Silver Leaf Jasper, Smoky Amethyst, Smoky Elestial Quartz, Tantalite, Thunder Egg, Valentinite and Stibnite, Xenotine

Psychic vampirism, block: Actinolite, Ammolite, Apple Aura Quartz, Banded Agate, Gaspeite, Green Aventurine, Green Fluorite, Iridescent Pyrite, Jade, Jet, Labradorite, Lemurian Aquitane Calcite, Nunderite, Prasiolite, Tantalite, Xenotine

Psychological integration: Graphic Smoky Quartz, Zebra Stone, Zircon

Psychological shadow, reveal: Agrellite, Azeztulite with Morganite, Champagne Aura Quartz, Covellite, Day and Night Quartz, Lazulite, Lemurian Seed, Molybdenite, Nuummite, Phantom Quartz, Proustite, Shaman Quartz, Smoky Elestial Quartz, Voegesite. *Chakra:* solar plexus

– Q –

Questionable channellings, discern truth of: Agate, Amazonite, Aquamarine, Celestite, Charoite, Danburite, Green Kyanite, Iolite, Lapis Lazuli, Obsidian, Pietersite, Sapphire, Scheelite, Tiger's Eye

– R –

Radiation, counteract: Amber, Aventurine, Black Tourmaline, Boron, Cerussite, Chlorite Quartz, Cinnabar, Colemanite, Covellite, Crocoite, Galena (wash hands after use, make essence by indirect method), Graphic Smoky Quartz, Hackmanite, Herkimer Diamond, Jasper, Kernite, Klinoptilolith, Kunzite, Malachite (use as polished stone, make essence by indirect method), Morion, Orgonite, Ouro Verde, Quartz, Rainbow Covellite, Reinerite, Rutilated Quartz, Shungite, Smoky Elestial, Smoky Elestial Quartz, Smoky Quartz, Sodalite, Star Sapphire, Stibnite, Tantalite, Tektite, Torbernite, Uranophane, Velvet Malachite (under supervision), Yellow Kunzite. *Chakra:* earth star, base, higher heart. Place stones around source.

Radon gas: Boron, Chlorite Quartz, Covellite, Danburite, Diaspore, Eye of the Storm (rough form), Graphic Smoky Quartz, Halite, Herkimer Diamond, Klinoptilolith, Libyan Gold Tektite, Malachite, Morion Quartz, Ouro Verde, Pumice, Shungite, Smoky Elestial Quartz, Smoky Quartz, Sodalite, Tektite, Torbernite, Yellow Kunzite.

Place stones around source or wear continuously.

Reclaim power: Brandenberg Amethyst, Eilat Stone, Empowerite, Leopardskin Jasper, Nuummite, Owyhee Blue Opal, Rainbow Mayanite, Sceptre Quartz, Shiva Lingam, Smoky Elestial Quartz, Tinguaite. *Chakra:* past life, base

Reconciliation: Afghanite, Chinese Red Quartz, Pink Lazurine, Rose Quartz, Ruby Lavender Quartz. *Chakra:* heart seed

Repair, assist body to: Aegerine, Bixbite, Brandenberg Amethyst, Celestial Quartz, Molybdenite, Quantum Quattro Rutile with Hematite, Shungite, Zoisite. *Chakra:* dantien

Restraint, emotional or mental: Idocrase. *Chakra:* past life, heart

Retrieval, child or soul parts: Anandalite, Fulgarite, Khutnohorite, Tangerose, Youngite. *Chakra:* causal vortex, past life

Retrieve soul parts left at previous death: Lemurian Seed, Selenite, Smoky Spirit Quartz. *Chakra:* causal vortex, past life

– S –

Sabotage: Larimar, Lemurian Aquitane Calcite, Mohawkite, Scapolite, Scheelite, Tourmalinated Quartz, Turquoise

Sacral chakra: Amber, Amphibole, Bastnasite, Black Opal, Blue Jasper, Blue-green Fluorite, Blue-green Turquoise, Bumble Bee Jasper, Carnelian, Chinese Red Quartz, Citrine, Clinohumite, Golden and iron-coated Green Ridge Quartz, Golden Healer Quartz, Keyiapo, Limonite, Mahogany Obsidian, Orange Calcite, Orange Carnelian, Orange Kyanite, Orange Zincite, Realgar and Orpiment, Red Amethyst, Red Jasper, Red/Orange Zincite, Tangerose, Topaz, Triplite, Vanadinite (wash hands after use, make essence by indirect method). *Chakra:* sacral/navel

> **balance and align:** Anandalite, Celestobarite, Golden Healer Quartz, Green Ridge Quartz
>
> **spin too rapid/stuck open:** Amber, Black Opal, Blue-green Fluorite, Blue-green Turquoise
>
> **spin too sluggish/stuck closed:** Carnelian, Orange Zincite, Topaz, Triplite

Safe passage: Aquamarine *(when at sea)*, Cerussite, Desert Rose, Emerald, Moonstone *(when at sea)*, Orange Zircon, Tourmalinated Quartz, Turquoise, Yellow Jasper

Scapegoating behaviour: Champagne Aura Quartz, Mohawkite, Scapolite, Smoky Amethyst

Seasonal affective disorder: Carnelian, Citrine, Kunzite, Sunshine Aura Quartz, Sunstone, Topaz, Triplite. Wear continuously.

Security issues: Chinese Red Quartz, Nzuri Moyo. *Chakra:* base

   emotional: Mangano Vesuvianite, Oceanite, Tugtupite. *Chakra:* base, dantien, solar plexus

   letting go of: Axinite, Scheelite. *Chakra:* base, dantien

Self-defeating programs: Desert Rose, Drusy Quartz, Kinoite, Nuummite, Paraiba Tourmaline, Quantum Quattro, Strawberry Quartz

Self-hatred (combating): Blizzard Stone, Luvulite, Quantum Quattro, Rose Quartz, Spirit Quartz, Sugilite, Tugtupite. *Chakra:* base

Self-sabotaging behaviour: Agrellite, Quantum Quattro, Scapolite and see Sabotage, above.

Shamanic journeys: see Travel page 347

Shield yourself: Black Tourmaline, Healer's Gold, Nuummite, Polychrome Jasper, Pyrite, Shieldite, Shungite, Smoky Quartz. *Chakra:* higher heart

Sick building syndrome: Amber, Aragonite, Aventurine, Black Tourmaline, Celtic Quartz, Chlorite Quartz, Covellite, Fire Agate, Galena (wash hands after use), Graphic Smoky Quartz, Hackmanite, Halite, Hanksite, Lepidolite, Marble, Morion, Orgonite, Preseli Bluestone, Pumice, Quartz, Rose Quartz, Selenite, Shieldite, Shungite, Smoky Elestial Quartz, Smoky Quartz, Sodalite, Tourmaline, Trummer Jasper. Place around building, zigzag in room or wear constantly.

Solar plexus chakra: Calcite, Citrine, Citrine Herkimer, Golden Azeztulite, Golden Beryl, Golden Calcite, Golden

Coracalcite, Golden Danburite, Golden Enhydro, Golden Healer, Golden Labradorite (Bytownite), Green Chrysoprase, Green Prehnite, Green Ridge Quartz, Jasper, Libyan Glass Tektite, Light Green Hiddenite, Malachite (use as polished stone, make essence by indirect method), Obsidian, Rainbow Obsidian, Rhodochrosite, Rhodozite, Smoky Quartz, Sunstone, Tangerine Aura Quartz, Tangerine Dream Lemurian Seed, Tiger's Eye, Yellow Tourmaline, Yellow Zincite

balance and align: Anandalite, Citrine, Lemurian Seed

spin too rapid/stuck open: Calcite, Light Green Hiddenite, Malachite, Rainbow Obsidian, Smoky Quartz

spin too sluggish/stuck closed: Golden Calcite, Golden Danburite, Tangerine Aura Quartz, Yellow Labradorite (Bytownite)

Soma chakra: Afghanite, Amechlorite, Angelinite, Angel's Wing Calcite, Astraline, Auralite 23, Azeztulite, Banded Agate, Brandenberg Amethyst, Champagne Aura Quartz, Crystal Cap Amethyst, Diaspore (Zultanite), Faden Quartz, Fire and Ice, Holly Agate, Ilmenite, Isis Calcite, Lemurian Aquatine Calcite, Merkabite Calcite, Natrolite, Nuummite, Owyhee Blue Opal, Pentagonite, Petalite, Phantom Calcite, Phenacite on Fluorite, Preseli Bluestone, Red Amethyst, Sacred Scribe, Satyaloka and Satyamani Quartz, Scolecite, Sedona Stone, Shaman Quartz, Stellar Beam Calcite, Trigonic Quartz, Violane, Z-stone. *Chakra:* soma, mid-hairline

balance and align: Bytownite, Diaspore, Stellar Beam Calcite, Violane

spin too rapid/stuck open: Isis Calcite, Pinky-beige Ussingite, Sedona Stone, Shaman Quartz, White Banded Agate

spin too sluggish/stuck closed: Banded Agate, Diaspore, Nuummite, Preseli Bluestone

Sorcery, protect against: Nuummite, Purpurite, Shamanite, Tourmaline

Soul cleanser: Anandalite, Black Kyanite, Brandenberg Amethyst, Chinese Chromium Quartz, Chrysotile in Serpentine, Golden Danburite, Golden Healer, Khutnohorite, Prehnite with Epidote, Rutile with Hematite, Selenite, Smoky Cathedral Quartz, Smoky Elestial Quartz

Soul contracts, recognition and release: Agate, Black Kyanite, Boli Stone, Brandenberg Amethyst, Charoite, Dumortierite, Flint, Gabbro, Green Aventurine, Kakortokite, Leopardskin Jasper, Pyrophyllite, Rainbow Mayanite, Red Amethyst, Wind Fossil Agate, Wulfenite. *Chakra:* past life, higher crown, causal vortex

Soul encrustations: Ethiopian Opal

Soul fragmentation: Anandalite, Angel's Wing Calcite, Brandenberg, Selenite. *Chakra:* past life

Soul healing: Amphibole, Black Kyanite, Blue Aragonite, Brandenberg Amethyst, Cassiterite, Ethiopian Opal, Fiskenaesset Ruby, Golden Healer, Khutnohorite, Marble, Nuummite, Pink Lazurine, Porphyrite (Chinese Letter Stone), Preseli Bluestone, Ruby Lavender Quartz,

Trigonic Quartz

Soul imperatives: Nirvana Quartz, Porphyrite (Chinese Letter Stone), Tantalite

Soul memory: Amphibole, Anandalite, Brandenberg Amethyst, Cacoxenite, Datolite, Trigonic Quartz

Soul retrieval: Amethyst Herkimer, Anandalite, Blue Euclase, Brandenberg Amethyst, Epidote, Faden Quartz, Flint, Fulgarite, Gaspeite, Herkimer Diamond, Khutnohorite, Kunzite, Kyanite, Lemurian Seed, Mount Shasta Opal, Nuummite, Preseli Bluestone, Rainbow Mayanite, Shiva Shells, Smithsonite, Smoky Amethyst, Smoky Brandenberg, Snakeskin Agate, Tangerine Quartz, Tangerose, Tibetan Quartz, Trigonic, Youngite. *Chakra:* higher heart, third eye, soma, heart seed and tap over points shown on page 127.

Soul splits: Trigonic Quartz, Twin Crystals, and see Soul retrieval above

Soul star chakra: Afghanite, Ajoite, Amethyst Elestial, Amphibole, Anandalite, Angel's Wing Calcite, Apophyllite, Astraline, Auralite 23, Azeztulite, Blue Flint, Brandenberg Amethyst, Celestite, Celestobarite, Chevron Amethyst, Citrine, Danburite, Dianite, Diaspore (Zultanite), Elestial Quartz, Fire and Ice, Fire and Ice and Nirvana Quartz, Golden Enhydro Herkimer, Golden Himalayan Azeztulite, Green Ridge Quartz, Hematite, Herkimer Diamond, Holly Agate, Keyiapo, Khutnohorite, Kunzite, Lapis Lazuli, Lavender Quartz, Merkabite Calcite, Muscovite, Natrolite, Novaculite, Nuummite, Onyx, Orange River Quartz, Petalite,

Phenacite, Phenacite in Feldspar, Prophecy Stone, Purple Siberian Quartz, Purpurite, Quartz, Rainbow Mayanite, Rosophia, Satyamani and Satyaloka Quartz, Scolecite, Selenite, Shungite, Snowflake Obsidian, Spirit Quartz, Stellar Beam Calcite, Sugilite, Tangerine Aura Quartz, Tanzanite, Tanzine Aura Quartz, Titanite (Sphene), Trigonic Quartz, Vera Cruz Amethyst, Violane, White Elestial. *Chakra:* soul star, a foot or so above head

> **balance and align:** Anandalite, Vera Cruz Amethyst, Violane
>
> **spin too rapid/stuck open:** Celestobarite, Novaculite, Nuummite, Pinky-beige Ussingite, White, Rose or Smoky Elestial Quartz
>
> **spin too sluggish/stuck closed:** Golden Himalayan Azeztulite, Petalite, Phenacite, Rosophia

Spirit attachment: Aegerine, Avalonite, Blue Selenite, Brandenberg Amethyst, Brown Jasper, Celestobarite, Citrine Herkimer, Datolite, Fluorite, Halite, Herkimer Diamond, Iolite, Kunzite, Labradorite, Larimar, Laser Quartz, Marcasite, Petalite, Pyrolusite, Selenite wand, Shattuckite, Smoky Amethyst, Smoky Citrine, Smoky Elestial, Smoky Phantom Quartz, Spirit Quartz, Stibnite, Yellow Phantom Quartz. *Chakra:* soma chakra, solar plexus or heart

> **ascertain where or what attachment is:** Aegerine, Apophyllite, Blue (Indicolite) Tourmaline, Celestobarite, Chrysolite, Quartz with Mica. *Chakra:* third eye
>
> **release disembodied spirits attached to places:**

Larimar, Marcasite, Smoky Amethyst. Leave in the room or site (the effect is enhanced if you add Astral Clear or Z14).

release mental attachments: Aegerine, Blue Halite, Limonite, Pyrolusite, Smoky Amethyst, Yellow Phantom Quartz. *Chakra:* third eye, soma, causal vortex

releasing attachment: Aegerine, Amethyst, Avalonite, Blue Selenite, Brandenberg Amethyst, Brown Jasper, Celestobarite, Citrine Herkimer, Datolite, Fluorite, Halite, Herkimer Diamond, Iolite, Kunzite, Labradorite, Larimar, Laser Quartz, Marcasite, Petalite, Phantom Quartz, Pyrolusite, Selenite wand, Shattuckite, Smoky Citrine, Smoky Elestial, Smoky Quartz, Spirit Quartz, Stibnite, Yellow Phantom Quartz. *Chakra:* soma, solar plexus or heart

remove ancestral attachment: Brandenberg Amethyst, Cradle of Humankind, Datolite (attachment carried in the genes), Fairy Quartz, Rainforest Jasper, Smoky Elestial, Spirit Quartz. *Chakra:* soma chakra or solar plexus

remove disembodied spirits after channelling or other metaphysical activity: Banded Agate, Botswana Agate, Shattuckite. *Chakra:* third eye

remove 'implants': Dravite (Brown) Tourmaline, Flint, Rainbow Mayanite, Purple Tourmaline, Smoky Amethyst. Place over site.

repair aura after removal: Aegerine, Anandalite, Faden Quartz, Laser Quartz, Phantom Quartzes,

Quartz, Selenite, Stibnite

Spirit release: Nirvana Quartz and see Entity release page 292

Spiritual guidance: Amethyst, Anandalite, Astrophyllite, Azeztulite, Azurite, Dumortierite, Indicolite Quartz, Kyanite, Lapis Lazuli, Mentor formation, Moldavite, Orange Calcite, Petalite, Phenacite, Pink Phantom Quartz, Smoky Amethyst, Smoky Elestial, Spirit Quartz, Super 7, Tanzanite, Tanzine Aura Quartz, Vivianite

Spiritual protection: see Protection page 324

Spleen chakra: Amber, Aventurine, Bloodstone, Carnelian, Chlorite Quartz, Emerald, Eye of the Storm, Fire Opal, Flint, Gaspeite, Green Aventurine, Green Fluorite, Jade, Orange River Quartz, Prasiolite, Rhodochrosite, Rhodonite, Ruby, Tugtupite, Zircon. *Chakra:* under left armpit

   balance and align: Charoite, Emerald, Eye of the Storm, Flint, Green Aventurine, Tugtupite

   clear attachments and hooks: Aventurine, Chert, Flint, Gaspeite, Jade, Jasper, Lemurian Seed

   right armpit: Bloodstone, Eye of the Storm, Gaspeite, Triplite, Tugtupite

   spin too rapid/stuck open: Amber, Aventurine, Chlorite Quartz, Eye of the Storm, Flint, Gaspeite, Green Fluorite, Jade, Prasiolite, Tugtupite

   spin too sluggish/stuck closed: Fire Opal, Orange River Quartz, Rhodonite, Ruby, Topaz

Stagnant energy, disperse: Black Tourmaline, Calcite, Chlorite Quartz, Chrome Diopside, Citrine, Clear Topaz,

Eye of the Storm, Garnet in Quartz, Golden Healer, Orgonite, Poppy Jasper, Quartz, Ruby Lavender Quartz, Sedona Stone, Selenite, Shaman Quartz, Smoky Elestial Quartz, Smoky Quartz, Tantalite, Triplite, and see Negative energy page 316. *Chakra:* base, dantien

Stale hotel room: Anandalite, Quartz with Petaltone Z14 or Clear2Light essence, Selenite

Stellar gateway chakra: Afghanite, Ajoite, Amethyst Elestial, Amphibole, Anandalite™, Angelinite, Angel's Wing Calcite, Apophyllite, Astraline, Azeztulite, Brandenberg Amethyst, Celestite, Dianite, Diaspore (Zultanite), Elestial Quartz, Fire and Ice, Golden Himalayan Azeztulite, Golden Selenite, Green Ridge Quartz, Holly Agate, Ice Quartz, Kunzite, Merkabite Calcite, Moldavite, Nirvana Quartz, Novaculite, Petalite, Phenacite, Purpurite, Stellar Beam Calcite, Titanite (Sphene), Trigonic Quartz, White Elestial Quartz. *Chakra:* arm's length above head

> **balance and align:** Ajoite, Amethyst Elestial, Anandalite, Brandenberg Amethyst, Kunzite
>
> **spin too rapid/stuck open:** Amphibole Quartz, Ice Quartz, Merkabite Calcite, Pinky-beige Ussingite, Purpurite
>
> **spin too sluggish/stuck closed:** Angel's Wing Calcite, Diaspore, Phenacite

Stress: Amber, Amethyst, Aquamarine, Aventurine, Beryl, Brandenberg Amethyst, Charoite, Dioptase, Eye of the Storm, Galaxyite, Golden Healer Quartz, Graphic Smoky Quartz, Green Aventurine, Herkimer Diamond,

Jade, Jasper, Labradorite, Lapis Lazuli, Magnetite, Marble, Petalite, Quantum Quattro, Que Sera, Rhodonite, Richterite, Rose Quartz, Serpentine, Shungite, Siberian Quartz, Smoky Quartz, Sodalite, Vera Cruz Amethyst

Stuck souls and inappropriate 'crystal mentors': Aegerine, Anandalite, Banded Agate, Candle Quartz, Flint, Jet, Quartz, Rainbow Mayanite, Rose Quartz, Shattuckite, Smoky Amethyst, Smoky Amethyst Brandenberg, Spirit Quartz, Stibnite, Super 7. *Chakra:* soma, third eye, causal vortex (or place in environment)

Study/home office: Amethyst, Ammolite, Fluorite, Jade, Pyrite, Sodalite

Subconscious blocks: Lepidocrocite, Molybdenite in Quartz, Smoky Elestial Quartz, Smoky Spirit Quartz. *Chakra:* dantien, soul star, stellar gateway, causal vortex, third eye, soma

Subtle energy bodies:

    ancestral: Ancestralite, Anthrophyllite, Blue Holly Agate, Brandenberg Amethyst, Bumble Bee Jasper, Candle Quartz, Catlinite, Cradle of Humankind, Datolite, Eclipse Stone, Fairy Quartz, Golden Healer, Icicle Calcite, Ilmenite, Jade, Kambaba Jasper, Lemurian Aquatine Calcite, Mohawkite, Peanut Wood, Petrified Wood, Porphyrite, Prasiolite, Rainbow Mayanite, Rainforest Jasper, Shaman Quartz, Smoky Elestial Quartz, Spirit Quartz, Starseed, Stromatolite. *Chakra:* soul star, past life, alta major, causal vortex, higher heart, earth star, Gaia gateway

    emotional: Apache Tear, Black Moonstone, Blue

Moonstone, Botswana (Banded) Agate, Brandenberg Amethyst, Calcite, Danburite, Golden Healer, Icicle Calcite, Kunzite, Lepidolite, Mangano Calcite, Moonstone, Pink Moonstone, Pink Petalite, Rainbow Mayanite, Rainbow Moonstone, Rainbow Obsidian, Rhodochrosite, Rhodonite, Rose Elestial Quartz, Rose Quartz, Rubellite, Selenite, Tourmalinated Quartz, Tugtupite, Watermelon Tourmaline. *Chakra:* solar plexus, three-chambered heart, sacral and base chakras, knees and feet.

etheric: Andescine Labradorite, Angelinite, Astraline, Brandenberg Amethyst, Chlorite Quartz, Chrysotile, Cradle of Humankind, Datolite, Elestial Quartz, Ethiopian Opal, Eye of the Storm, Flint, Girasol, Golden Healer, Icicle Calcite, Keyiapo, Khutnohorite, Lemurian Aquitane Calcite, Poldervaarite, Pollucite, Quantum Quattro, Que Sera, Rainbow Mayanite, Rhodozite, Ruby Lavender Quartz, Sanda Rosa Azeztulite, Scheelite, Selenite, Shaman Quartz, Shungite, Stellar Beam Calcite, Tangerine Dream Lemurian, Tantalite. *Chakra:* 7 traditional chakras, plus soma, past life, alta major, causal vortex

karmic/karmic blueprint: Ammolite, Ammonite, Ancestralite, Brandenberg Amethyst, Cloudy Quartz, Cradle of Humankind, Crinoidal Limestone, Datolite, Dumortierite, Flint, Kambaba Jasper, Keyiapo, Khutnohorite, Lemurian Seed, Nirvana Quartz, Rainbow Mayanite, Rhodozite, Ruby Lavender Quartz, Sanda Rosa Azeztulite, Scheelite, Shaman

Quartz, Shungite, Stromatolite, Titanite (Sphene) and see page 309. *Chakra:* past life, alta major, causal vortex, soma, knee and earth star

lightbody: Agnitite™, Anandalite™, Angel's Wing Calcite, Blue Moonstone, Brandenberg Amethyst, Chlorite Brandenberg, Eklogite, Erythrite, Golden Coracalcite, Golden Healer Quartz, Golden Himalayan Azeztulite, Hackmanite, Himalayan Gold Azeztulite™, Lemurian Seed, Lilac-purple Coquimbite, Madagascan Red 'Celestial Quartz', Mahogany Sheen Obsidian, Merkabite Calcite, Natrolite, Nirvana Quartz, Opal Aura Quartz, Phantom Calcite, Phenacite, Pink Lemurian, Prophecy Stone, Rainbow Mayanite, Red Amethyst, Rutilated Quartz (Angel Hair), Rutile with Hematite, Satyaloka Quartz, Satyamani Quartz, Scolecite, Spirit Quartz, Sugar Blade Quartz, Tangerine Dream Lemurian, Tiffany Stone, Trigonic Quartz, Tugtupite, Vera Cruz Amethyst, Violet Ussingite. *Chakra:* soma, soul star, stellar gateway, Gaia gateway, alta major, causal vortex

mental: Amechlorite, Amethyst, Arfvedsonite, Auralite 23, Brandenberg Amethyst, Celadonite, Chlorite Brandenberg, Crystal Cap Amethyst, Dumortierite, Fluorite, Lemurian Seed, Merkabite Calcite, Nuummite, Owyhee Blue Opal, Rainbow Covellite, Rainbow Mayanite, Sapphire, Scheelite, Scolecite, Sodalite, Sugilite, Vera Cruz Amethyst. *Chakra:* third eye, soma, alta major, causal vortex

physical, subtle: Amechlorite, Anandalite, Ancestralite, Bloodstone, Brandenberg Amethyst, Carnelian, Cradle of Humankind, Dumortierite, Eilat Stone, Eklogite, Flint, Hematite, Kambaba Jasper, Madagascan Red 'Celestial Quartz', Quantum Quattro, Que Sera, Rainbow Mayanite, Red Amethyst, Stromatolite. *Chakras:* base, sacral, dantien, earth star

planetary: Aswan Granite, Brandenberg Amethyst, Celtic Quartz, Charoite, Lapis Lazuli, Libyan Gold Tektite, Moldavite, Nebula Stone, Preseli Bluestone, Rainbow Mayanite, Starseed Quartz, Tektite, Trigonic. *Chakra:* past life, alta major, causal vortex, soma, stellar and Gaia gateway chakras

spiritual: Anandalite, Azeztulite, Brandenberg Amethyst, Golden Quartz, Golden Herkimer Diamond, Green Ridge Quartz, Larimar, Lemurian Seed, Nirvana Quartz, Phenacite, Rainbow Mayanite, Shaman Quartz, Trigonic Amethyst, Trigonic Quartz. *Chakra:* past life, soul star, stellar gateway, alta major, causal vortex

Sudden energy drain: Agate, Apache Tear, Black Tourmaline, Carnelian, Green Aventurine, Green Fluorite, Jade, Labradorite, Polychrome Jasper, Red Jasper, Shungite, Triplite

Survival instincts: Ammolite, Kimberlite, Thunder Egg. *Chakra:* base

– T –

Taking on other people's feelings or conditions: Black Tourmaline, Brochantite, Healer's Gold, Iridescent Pyrite, Labradorite, Lemurian Jade, Mohawkite. *Chakra:* solar plexus, spleen

Third eye (brow) chakra: Afghanite, Ajo Quartz, Ajoite, Amber, Amechlorite, Amethyst, Ammolite, Amphibole Quartz, Angelite, Apophyllite, Aquamarine, Axinite, Azurite, Black Moonstone, Blue Calcite, Blue Kyanite, Blue Lace Agate, Blue Obsidian, Blue Selenite, Blue Topaz, Blue Tourmaline, Bytownite (Yellow Labradorite), Cacoxenite, Cavansite, Champagne Aura Quartz, Diaspore, Electric-blue Obsidian, Eye of the Storm, Garnet, Glaucophane, Golden Himalayan Azeztulite, Herderite, Herkimer Diamond, Holly Agate, Howlite, Indigo Auram, Iolite, Kunzite, Labradorite, Lapis Lazuli, Lavender-purple Opal, Lazulite, Lepidolite, Libyan Gold Tektite, Malachite with Azurite (use as polished stone, make essence by indirect method), Moldavite, Pietersite, Purple Fluorite, Rhomboid Selenite, Sapphire, Serpentine in Obsidian, Sodalite, Spectrolite, Stilbite, Sugilite, Tangerine Aura Quartz, Turquoise, Unakite, Yellow Labradorite (Bytownite). *Chakra:* above and between eyebrows

> **balance and align:** Anandalite, Sugilite
> **spin too rapid/stuck open:** Diaspore, Iolite, Lavender-purple Opal, Pietersite, Serpentine in Obsidian, Sodalite, Sugilite

spin too sluggish/stuck closed: Apophyllite, Azurite, Banded Agate, Diaspore, Herkimer Diamond, Optical Calcite, Rhomboid Calcite, Rhomboid Selenite, Royal Blue Sapphire, Tanzine Aura Quartz, Yellow Labradorite (Bytownite)

Thought form, disperse: Aegerine, Amethyst, Azurite, Blue Selenite, Blue Tourmaline, Brown Jasper, Celestobarite, Citrine, Citrine Herkimer, Clear Kunzite, Firework Obsidian, Herkimer, Herkimer Diamond, Iolite, Kunzite, Labradorite, Nuummite, Pyrolusite, Rainbow Mayanite, Scolecite, Smoky Amethyst, Smoky Citrine, Spectrolite, Stibnite. *Chakra:* dowse to see which of the chakras around the head is affected.

Throat chakra: Ajo Quartz, Ajoite, Amber, Amethyst, Aquamarine, Astraline, Azurite, Blue Chalcedony, Blue Kyanite, Blue Lace Agate, Blue Obsidian, Blue Quartz, Blue Topaz, Blue Tourmaline, Chalcanthite, Chrysocolla, Chrysotile, Eye of the Storm, Glaucophane, Green Ridge Quartz, Indicolite Quartz, Kunzite, Lapis Lazuli, Lepidolite, Moldavite, Paraiba Tourmaline, Sugilite, Turquoise. Place over throat.

> **balance and align:** Anandalite, Blue Chalcedony, Blue Lace Agate, Blue Topaz, Indicolite Quartz, Sapphire
> **spin too rapid/stuck open:** Black Sapphire, Lepidolite, Paraiba Tourmaline, Sugilite, Turquoise
> **spin too sluggish/stuck closed:** Chrysocolla, Lapis Lazuli, Moldavite, Turquoise

Tie cutting: see Cord cutting, page 277

Toxic earth meridians: Amber, Chlorite Quartz, Granite,

Graphic Smoky Quartz, Kambaba Jasper, Marble, Mohawkite, Orgonite, Preseli Bluestone, Quartz, Shieldite, Shungite, Smoky Elestial Quartz, Snakeskin Pyrite, Sodalite, Valentinite and Stibnite

Toxicity: Amber, Arsenopyrite, Champagne Aura Quartz, Chlorite Quartz, Green Jasper, Halite, Hanksite, Klinoptilolith, Morion Quartz, Orgonite, Rutilated Quartz, Shieldite, Smoky Elestial Quartz, Smoky Quartz, Snakeskin Pyrite, Sodalite, Sunshine Aura Quartz, Tourmalinated Quartz, Valentinite and Stibnite. *Chakra:* dantien, earth, spleen. Place in environment

Toxins: see Detoxification page 281. *Chakra:* earth star, spleen

> **disperse:** Actinolite, Aegerine, Ametrine, Banded Agate, Barite, Blue Quartz, Celestite, Celestobarite, Champagne Aura Quartz, Chinese Chromium Quartz, Chlorite Quartz, Chrysanthemum Stone, Conichalcite, Covellite, Danburite with Chlorite, Eilat Stone, Epidote, Eye of the Storm, Fairy Quartz, Fiskenaesset Ruby, Golden Danburite, Halite, Hanksite, Huebnerite, Iolite, Leopardskin Serpentine, Morion, Ocean Jasper, Orgonite, Pearl Spa Dolomite, Poppy Jasper, Pumice, Pyrite in Quartz, Quantum Quattro, Seraphinite, Serpentine, Shieldite, Smoky Elestial Quartz, Smoky Herkimer, Snakeskin Pyrite, Sodalite, Spirit Quartz, Yellow Apatite. *Chakra:* base, earth star, dantien, spleen, solar plexus

> **disperse from environment:** Chlorite Quartz, Chrysanthemum Stone, Orgonite, Shieldite, Shungite,

Sodalite

remove: Ametrine, Celestite, Chlorite Quartz, Iolite, Moss Agate, Orgonite, Serpentine, Shieldite, Shungite, Sodalite, Yellow Apatite. *Chakra*: base, earth, spleen, solar plexus

strengthen resistance to: Beryl, Eye of the Storm, Klinoptilolith, Ocean Jasper, Pyrite in Quartz, Shungite. *Chakra*: base, earth star, dantien, spleen, solar plexus

Trauma: Ammolite, Blue Euclase, Bornite, Brandenberg Amethyst, Cathedral Quartz, Cavansite, Dumortierite, Empowerite, Epidote, Faden Quartz, Fulgarite, Gaia Stone, Garnet in Quartz, Goethite, Golden Healer, Green Diopside, Green Ridge Quartz, Guardian Stone, Kimberlite, Mangano Vesuvianite, Novaculite with Nuummite, Ocean Blue Jasper, Oregon Opal, Peach Selenite, Peanut Wood, Prasiolite, Richterite, Ruby Lavender Quartz, Scapolite, Sea Sediment Jasper, Smoky Elestial, Spirit Quartz, Tantalite, Victorite, Wavellite, Youngite. *Chakra:* solar plexus. (Or wear constantly.)

Travel, protection during: Amethyst, Aquamarine, Cerussite, Chalcedony, Eye of the Storm (Judy's Jasper), Garnet, Herkimer Diamond, Jet, Malachite, Moldavite, Moonstone, Nuummite, Orgonite, Petalite, Preseli Bluestone, Rainbow Moonstone, Rhodonite, Shieldite, Shungite, Smoky Quartz, Tiger's Eye, Turquoise, Yellow Jasper. Keep stone in pocket or wear around neck.

car: Blue Chalcedony, Carnelian, Nuummite, Preseli Bluestone, Rhodonite, Shungite, Tiger's Eye

on horseback: Turquoise

on land: Turquoise

on sea: Aquamarine, Moonstone

plane: Blue Chalcedony, Flint, Preseli Bluestone, Shungite

shamanic journeys: Ametrine, Ammolite, Apache Tear, Astrophyllite, Azurite, Black Kyanite, Boji Stones, Bronzite, Celestobarite, Chevron Amethyst, Desert Rose, Dumortierite, Flint, Gaia Stone, Iolite, Jasper, Kunzite, Labradorite, Lapis Lazuli, Leopardskin Agate/Jasper/Serpentine, Menalite, Novaculite, Nuummite, Obsidian, Pietersite, Preseli Bluestone, Rhyolite, Rutilated Quartz, Shungite, Smoky Amethyst, Smoky Quartz, Snakeskin Agate, Stibnite, Tourmalinated Quartz, Tourmaline, Turquoise. *Chakra:* Hold or place over soma chakra and third eye. And see Safe passage page 330.

– U –

Unacceptable thoughts and feelings, release: Golden Healer, Scolecite, Vivianite. *Chakra:* solar plexus, third eye

Unconditional love: Astraline, Cobalto Calcite, Erythrite, Luvulite, Mangano Calcite, Rhodochrosite, Rhodonite, Rose Quartz, Sugilite, Tangerose, Tugtupite. *Chakra:* higher heart. (Wear continuously or place over higher heart.)

Unconditional self-love: Citrine, Emerald, Erythrite, Luvulite, Mangano Calcite, Pink Calcite, Rose Quartz, Sugilite, Tugtupite. *Chakra:* heart

Uncursing: Black Tourmaline, Novaculite, Nuummite, Stibnite, Tourmalinated Quartz, and see Curses page 278

Undead, protection against: Black Sapphire, Chalcedony, Silver settings

Undue mental influence/attachments: Aegerine, Blue Halite, Celtic Quartz, Limonite, Pyrolusite, Shungite, Smoky Amethyst, Yellow Phantom Quartz

Ungroundedness: Aztee, Basalt, Boji Stones, Celestobarite, Chlorite Quartz, Dragon Stone, Empowerite, Flint, Granite, Graphic Smoky Quartz (Zebra Stone), Hematite, Kambaba Jasper, Mohawkite, Peanut Wood, Petrified Wood, Polychrome Jasper, Proustite, Serpentine in Obsidian, Shell Jasper, Smoky Elestial Quartz, Steatite, Stromatolite. *Chakra:* earth star, base, dantien, Gaia gateway. Or place behind knees.

– V –

Vampirism of heart energy: Gaspeite, Green Aventurine, Greenlandite, Iridescent Pyrite, Jade, Lemurian Aquitane Calcite, Mohawkite, Nunderite, Tantalite, Xenotine. *Chakra:* solar plexus, heart, higher heart

Vampirism of spleen energy: Gaspeite, Green Aventurine, Green Fluorite, Iridescent Pyrite, Jade, Mohawkite, Nunderite, Tantalite, Xenotine. *Chakra:* spleen

Vibrational change, facilitate: Anandalite, Bismuth, Gabbro, Huebnerite, Lemurian Gold Opal, Lemurian Jade, Luxullianite, Montebrasite, Mtrolite, Nunderite, Rainbow Mayanite, Rosophia, Sanda Rosa Azeztulite, Snakeskin Pyrite, Sonora Sunrise, Trigonic Quartz. *Chakra:* higher heart, higher crown. Wear stones continuously, or keep within reach and hold frequently.

Victim mentality: Amblygonite, Brazilianite, Epidote, Green Ridge Quartz, Hematoid Calcite, Ice Quartz, Marcasite, Orange River Quartz, Rose Quartz, Smoky Lemurian Seed, Tugtupite with Nuummite, Zircon. *Chakra:* dantien

Violence, negate: Eye of the Storm (Judy's Jasper). *Chakra:* base (keep in environment)

Violence, protect against: Carnelian, Jet, Sardonyx, Turquoise

Viral infections: Cathedral Quartz, Himalayan Red Azeztulite, Proustite, Quantum Quattro, Rainforest Jasper, Shaman Quartz, Shungite, and see Antibacterial and antiviral page 260. *Chakra:* higher heart

Visualization: Amethyst, Annabergite, Apophyllite pyramid, Azurite, Blue or Rhomboid Calcite, Golden Labradorite (Bytownite), Lapis Lazuli, Prehnite, Selenite or Blue Selenite. *Chakra:* third eye

Vows and promises, release: Ancestralite, Brandenberg Amethyst, Dumortierite, Freedom Stone, Leopardskin Jasper, Pietersite, Pyrophyllite. *Chakra:* brow, soma, past life, causal vortex

– W –

Weak energy field: Celestobarite, Chlorite Quartz, Chrome Diopside, Orgonite, Poppy Jasper, Quantum Quattro, Que Sera, Sedona Stone. *Chakra:* hold between sacral and solar plexus

Weak muscles: Blue Moonstone, Magnetite

Weather sensitivity: Apricot Quartz, Avalonite, Chlorite Quartz, Golden Healer Quartz, Golden Pietersite, Khutnohorite, Quantum Quattro, Que Sera, Poppy Jasper, Shell Jasper, Shungite, Sillimanite, Silver Leaf Jasper, Trummer Jasper, Wonder Stone. *Chakra:* third eye

Wise mentor: Blue Chalcedony, Faden Quartz, Mentor Formation, Petalite, Selenite, Spirit Quartz, Tanzanite, Trigonic Quartz. *Chakra:* third eye, soma

Workplace harmonizers: Amber, Black Tourmaline, Clear Quartz, Eye of the Storm, Fluorite, Green Chlorite Quartz, Rose Quartz, Shungite, Siberian Green Quartz, Smoky Quartz, Turquoise

Wounds, imprints in etheric body: Ajoite, Ancestralite, Andean Blue Opal, Atlantasite, Bixbite, Cradle of Humankind, Diaspore (Zultanite), Flint, Gaia Stone, Golden Healer, Klinoptilolith, Lakelandite, Mookaite Jasper, Pumice, Quantum Quattro, Sceptre Quartz, Schalenblende, Seriphos Quartz, Shungite, Smoky Amethyst, Tibetan Black Spot Quartz, Youngite. *Chakra:* past life over site.

– X –

X-rays, prevent damage from: Amazonite, Aventurine, Black Moonstone, Chlorite Quartz, Herkimer Diamond, Lepidolite, Malachite, Malacolla, Orgonite, Shieldite, Shungite, Smoky Elestial Quartz, Smoky Herkimer, Smoky Quartz, Sodalite, Torbernite *(use under supervision)* and see Radiation page 328. Wear constantly, rub crystal essence over site, take crystal essence frequently.

– Y –

Yin-yang imbalances: Alunite, Dalmatian Stone, Day and Night Quartz, Eilat Stone, Morion, Poppy Jasper, Scheelite, Shiva Lingam, Strawberry Lemurian. *Chakra:* base, dantien

– Z –

Zest for life, restore: Bushman Red Cascade, Orange River Quartz, Poppy Jasper, Zebra Stone. *Chakra:* dantien
Zigzag layout: Amber, Black Tourmaline, Citrine, Flint, Golden Healer, Magnetite, Quartz, Selenite, Smoky Quartz

Footnotes

1. See *Crystal Prescriptions volume 3* for a comprehensive list of symptoms and effects and the research associated with this syndrome. Useful sites are included in the Resources guide.

2. See http://www.royalrife.com/powerlines.html, Peter Staheli, "Power Lines – not Radiation but Static Electricity Causes Diseases and Cancer".

3. http://themindunleashed.org/2014/01/scientific-proof-thoughts-intentions-can-alter-physical-world-around-us.html has video footage of the experiment.

4. See my *Book of Psychic Development* for details of 'Peter', a thought form created by a group of scientists that then went on to communicate with them through a medium.

5. *Thought-Forms*, Annie Besant and CW Leadbeater. Not the easiest of reads, but fascinating nonetheless. See http://www.gutenberg.org/files/16269/16269-h/16269-h.htm for a free, illustrated version.

Resources

Crystals

Crystals specially attuned for you by Judy Hall are available from: www.angeladditions.co.uk

In the US excellent crystals can be obtained from: www.exquisitecrystals.com

Essences

Petaltone cleansing and recharging essences: www.petaltone.co.uk or www.petaltone.com

Crystal Balance cleansing and recharging essences: www.crystalbalance.net

Green Man essences: www.greenmanshop.co.uk

Further reading

Hall, Judy:

Crystal Prescriptions volumes 1–4 (O-Books)

Crystal Wisdom Healing Oracle Kit (Watkins, 2016)

Good Vibrations (Flying Horse)

Crystal Skulls (Red Wheel/Weiser, October 2016)

Earth Blessings: Using Crystals for Personal Energy Clearing, Earth Healing and Environmental Enhancement (Watkins Publishing)

Crystals for Psychic Self-Protection (Hay House)
Crystal Bibles volumes 1–3 (Godsfield Press)
The Encyclopedia of Crystals (Hamlyn/Fair Winds Press)
Judy Hall's Book of Psychic Development (Flying Horse)
Crystals and Sacred Sites (Fair Winds Press/Quarto)
101 Power Crystals (Fair Winds Press/Quarto)
Crystal Healing Pack (Godsfield Press)

Crocker, Nicky, *What If It Was That Easy* [geopathic and EMF solutions]

Internet sources

Peter Staheli, "Power Lines – not Radiation but Static Electricity Causes Diseases and Cancer", http://www.royalrife.com/powerlines.html, accessed 21.2.2016

See "Measurement of the Human Biofield and Other Energetic Instruments", by Dr Beverly Rubik, Chapter 20, in Part Five, "Energetics and Spirituality" of *Mosby's Complementary and Alternative Medicine*, by Lyn Freeman http://www.faim.org/measurement-of-the-human-biofield-and-other-energetic-instruments for a useful overview of the human energy field and instruments that measure it.

The effects of chemical pollution: "The impact of chemical pollution on male reproductive health" http://ec.europa.eu/research/infocentre/article_en.cfm?id=/research/headlines/news/article_13_03_08_en.ht ml&artid=29333&item=Infocentre

Sick Building Syndrome, an overview:
http://www.nhs.uk/conditions/Sick-building-syndrome/Pages/Introduction.aspx

"Sick Building Syndrome: A Review Of The Evidence On Causes And Solutions", HSE:
www.hse.gov.uk/research/crr_pdf/1992/crr92042.pdf

"Sick Building Syndrome", BuildingEcology.com:
www.buildingecology.com/publications/ECA_Report4.pdf

"The sick building syndrome", by SM Joshi
http://www.ncbi.nlm.nih.gov/pmc/articles/PMC2796751/

Psychic assistance

College of Psychic Studies
16 Queensberry Place
London SW7 2EB
www.collegeofpsychicstudies.co.uk

School of Intuition and Healing
London Contact:
Phone: 0208-7782763
or 07875-225200

Telephone hours are 9am–7pm on Monday to Friday and 10am–5pm on Saturdays. Please do not phone outside these hours.

Cape Town contact:

072 5656072
(Cindy Holmes – Director)
082 5540554
(Penny Gaines – Administrator)

BOOKS

O-BOOKS

SPIRITUALITY

O is a symbol of the world, of oneness and unity; this
eye represents knowledge and insight. We publish titles
on general spirituality and living a spiritual life. We aim
to inform and help you on your own journey in this life.
If you have enjoyed this book, why not tell other readers
by posting a review on your preferred book site?

Recent bestsellers from O-Books are:

Heart of Tantric Sex
Diana Richardson
Revealing Eastern secrets of deep love and intimacy to
Western couples.
Paperback: 978-1-90381-637-0 ebook: 978-1-84694-637-0

Crystal Prescriptions
The A-Z guide to over 1,200 symptoms and their healing
crystals
Judy Hall
The first in the popular series of eight books, this handy
little guide is packed as tight as a pill-bottle with crystal
remedies for ailments.
Paperback: 978-1-90504-740-6 ebook: 978-1-84694-629-5

Take Me To Truth
Undoing the Ego
Nouk Sanchez, Tomas Vieira
The best-selling step-by-step book on shedding the Ego,
using the teachings of *A Course In Miracles*.
Paperback: 978-1-84694-050-7 ebook: 978-1-84694-654-7

The 7 Myths about Love...Actually!
The journey from your HEAD to the HEART of your SOUL
Mike George
Smashes all the myths about LOVE.
Paperback: 978-1-84694-288-4 ebook: 978-1-84694-682-0

365 Days of Wisdom
Daily Messages To Inspire You Through The Year
Dadi Janki
Daily messages which cool the mind, warm the heart
and guide you along your journey.
Paperback: 978-1-84694-863-3 ebook: 978-1-84694-864-0

Body of Wisdom
Women's Spiritual Power and How it Serves
Hilary Hart
Bringing together the dreams and experiences of women
across the world with today's most visionary spiritual
teachers.
Paperback: 978-1-78099-696-7 ebook: 978-1-78099-695-0

Dying to Be Free
From Enforced Secrecy to Near Death to True
Transformation
Hannah Robinson
After an unexpected accident and near-death
experience, Hannah Robinson found herself radically
transforming her life, while a remarkable new insight
altered her relationship with her father a practising
Catholic priest.
Paperback: 978-1-78535-254-6 ebook: 978-1-78535-255-3

The Ecology of the Soul
A Manual of Peace, Power and Personal Growth for Real
People in the Real World
Aidan Walker
Balance your own inner Ecology of the Soul to regain
your natural state of peace, power and wellbeing.
Paperback: 978-1-78279-850-7 ebook: 978-1-78279-849-1

Not I, Not other than I
The Life and Teachings of Russel Williams
Steve Taylor, Russel Williams
The miraculous life and inspiring teachings of one of the
World's greatest living Sages.
Paperback: 978-1-78279-729-6 ebook: 978-1-78279-728-9

On the Other Side of Love
A Woman's Unconventional Journey Towards Wisdom
Muriel Maufroy
When life has lost all meaning, what do you do?
Paperback: 978-1-78535-281-2 ebook: 978-1-78535-282-9

Practicing A Course In Miracles
A Translation of the Workbook in Plain Language and
With Mentoring Notes
Elizabeth A. Cronkhite
The practical second and third volumes of The Plain-
Language *A Course In Miracles*.
Paperback: 978-1-84694-403-1 ebook: 978-1-78099-072-9

Quantum Bliss

The Quantum Mechanics of Happiness, Abundance, and Health

George S. Mentz

Quantum Bliss is the breakthrough summary of success and spirituality secrets that customers have been waiting for.

Paperback: 978-1-78535-203-4 ebook: 978-1-78535-204-1

The Upside Down Mountain

Mags MacKean

A must-read for anyone weary of chasing success and happiness – one woman's inspirational journey swapping the uphill slog for the downhill slope.

Paperback: 978-1-78535-171-6 ebook: 978-1-78535-172-3

Your Personal Tuning Fork

The Endocrine System

Deborah Bates

Discover your body's health secret, the endocrine system, and 'twang' your way to sustainable health!

Paperback: 978-1-84694-503-8 ebook: 978-1-78099-697-4

Readers of ebooks can buy or view any of these
bestsellers by clicking on the live link in the title. Most
titles are published in paperback and as an ebook.
Paperbacks are available in traditional bookshops. Both
print and ebook formats are available online.

Find more titles and sign up to our readers' newsletter at
http://www.johnhuntpublishing.com/mind-body-spirit

Follow us on Facebook at
https://www.facebook.com/OBooks/